PSYCHIATRIC ILLNESS IN ADOLESCENCE

its psychopathology and prognosis

PSYCHIATRIC ILLNESS IN ADOLESCENCE

its psychopathology and prognosis

M. T. HASLAM
M.A., M.D.(Cantab.), M.R.C.P.(Glas.), M.R.C.Psych., D.P.M., D.M.J.
Consultant Psychiatrist, Clifton Hospital, York

BUTTERWORTHS
LONDON AND BOSTON

THE BUTTERWORTH GROUP

ENGLAND
Butterworth & Co (Publishers) Ltd
London: 88 Kingsway, WC2B 6AB

AUSTRALIA
Butterworths Pty Ltd
Sydney: 586 Pacific Highway, NSW 2067
Melbourne: 343 Little Collins Street, 3000
Brisbane: 240 Queen Street, 4000

CANADA
Butterworth & Co (Canada) Ltd
Toronto: 2265 Midland Avenue,
Scarborough, Ontario, M1P 4S1

NEW ZEALAND
Butterworths of New Zealand Ltd
Wellington: 26–28 Waring Taylor Street, 1

SOUTH AFRICA
Butterworth & Co (South Africa) (Pty) Ltd
Durban: 152–154 Gale Street

USA
Butterworth
161 Ash Street, Reading, Mass. 01867

First published 1975

Suggested U.D.C No. 616.89–053.7

ISBN 0 407 00019 4

Typeset, printed and bound in Great Britain by
REDWOOD BURN LIMITED
Trowbridge & Esher

CONTENTS

PREFACE

Western civilizations face particular problems in the upbringing of their children. This is principally the result of increasing industrialization with its tendency to produce a drift of population to the towns and a splitting up of family units.

In the old village communities it was rare for a child to need to be placed among strangers. There were always grandparents, aunts and neighbours to provide a continuity of care and security in all but the severest of crises.

In our present society of high-rise flats, enforced movement of workers due to industrial needs, and the consequent situation where a married couple and their child may live in a neighbourhood new to them, with grandparents sometimes hundreds of miles away in another town, separation experiences at an age critical to the child's development are increasingly common.

Bowlby (1951) was probably the first to publicize the possible deleterious effect on the growing child when at a critical age an episode of emotional deprivation occurred.

Although his publication for the World Health Organization is now some twenty-five years old, it is surprising that recognition of his findings has still to be made in some quarters, and appropriate action to ameliorate the possible consequences of separation experiences in children is still a matter with which some authorities make precious little attempt to deal. This is apparent in the policy with regard to parental access to children in hospital—still not entirely satisfactory in spite of such organizations as the National Association for the Welfare of Children in Hospital; the method of running some local authority children's homes; policies over fostering and adoption, and above all the education of parents or parents-to-be, which in the opinion of the author should start at school, and extend to both husband and wife in the antenatal clinics. Indeed even staff in the Social Services Departments, which have recently undergone reorganization, have not in the author's experience had their attention drawn as trainees to much of the work quoted in this book. They are thus unaware of the ever increasing accumulation of data from case studies, community surveys, and work with other animal species, all pointing to the possible damage which may be done, and which may lie dormant until the children have grown and sired or nutured children of their own.

One would hope that parents and prospective parents would think much more carefully of their responsibilities with regard to their offspring were they to be taught the already known facts on this subject at the appropriate time.

In this book a review of the literature on deprivation and separation experiences in children is made. Although some of Bowlby's work has been subject to modification, many well-known researchers including such workers as Rutter (1972) in the last few years, have established the importance of many of Bowlby's original concepts.

So many factors are likely to be of relevance in a child's early life both from the inheritance of intelligence and personality, and the acquisition, through experience of the environment, of modifications of these traits, that it is difficult to isolate and study particular problems exclusive of the rest. Since these factors will interact, but may have individual importance in the development of later emotional disablements, it is nevertheless important to make the attempt to do this, if the significance of these individual problems is to be elucidated.

The research presented in this book is an attempt to do this by picking out certain items of possible significance in the child's early history. By means of a retrospective and follow-up case study of one hundred adolescents (fifty with psychiatric difficulties, and fifty controls) some of these factors have been assessed, and their importance considered by means of quantifying the data and subjecting them to computer processing. Thus a correlation matrix can be obtained which will show how these factors may interrelate.

This has been made possible only with the generous help of those who are acknowledged, and many others, not least the one hundred adolescents and their relatives who generously gave of their time in order to assist the author in his studies.

M.T.H.

ACKNOWLEDGEMENTS

I would like to thank the following persons for their kind and helpful assistance over various aspects of the preparation of this book.

Professor Martin Roth, Dr. D. W. K. Kay, and Dr. J. P. Child for their helpful guidance and assistance in the collection of cases admitted to their departments.

The staff operating the Holerith punch-card sorter at Newcastle General Hospital, for assisting with this aspect of the study.

The staff of the Casualty Department, the Royal Victoria Infirmary, Newcastle upon Tyne, for their help in the collection of a control group.

The staff of the M.R.C. unit, Framlington Place, and in particular Helena Foster for her help in getting the data on to tape and obtaining the correlation matrices at the computer laboratory.

Particularly I would like to thank Miss Maureen Hudson for her help and for the typing of the manuscripts for this book, a task which has required much patience.

Finally, I would like to thank my wife for her help with many aspects of the interpretation of data, which meant giving up many evenings of her time.

I

INTRODUCTION AND HISTORICAL SURVEY

Adolescence is a critical period in the development of many psychiatric illnesses, yet as a group adolescents have been poorly catered for in psychiatric practice in this country. Diagnosis is notoriously unreliable in this age group, and prognostic indicators difficult to define. Many widely differing views are put forward as to the importance of early environmental happenings in the subsequent development of psychiatric disturbance, and it would appear that the period of adolescence is an ideal time to consider aspects of psychopathology, since information should still be readily available in the majority of cases from parents, concerning early events in the patient's life. Furthermore it is in adolescence that many of the disturbances which may develop will begin to show themselves. It is also an important period in that the personality is not yet entirely matured. Some modification may thus still be effected and the damage righted before the maturity of adulthood renders it too late, reversal being less possible once patterns of behaviour have become too rigidly fixed.

OUTLINE OF THE SIZE OF THE PROBLEM

Boyd (1967), discussing the problem of adolescence states that the admission rate of young people to our mental hospitals, from a steady level over several years of about 1500 first admissions in the age group 10–19, has shown an impressive rise to over 4500 in 1964, with a total of well over 7000 admissions. In December 1963, a census of this age group resident in mental hospitals totalled 1350 which represented 28 beds per million population. There has been an alarming increase in juvenile crime in the last nine years in the age group 14–20. The suicide rate, having been 28 per million since 1945, had increased to 43 per million by 1965; in the under 20 age group there were no known heroin addicts up to 1959 but in 1965 there were 134. In January 1964, the Ministry of Health stated that there were then only 157 psychiatric beds for adolescents, in seven special units. This represented slightly over three beds per million population. By 1969 there were ten adolescent units in England and Wales with about 200 beds, which provided only four beds per million of the population. With the accommodation at present proposed a total of about 12 beds per million will be provided eventually. The Ministry of Health recommendations would have meant a total of 1100 beds especially allocated. The survey performed by the National Association for Mental Health (1966) showed that eight regions had no special beds for adolescents at all.

In contrast, in the United States, according to the *American Journal of Psychiatry* (1967) out-patient psychiatric clinics see more adolescents than any other decade—a quarter of all clinic patients. In-patients had increased by 325 per cent in the period 1950–1963.

In Western Germany there were by 1966 two clinics in child psychiatry, with clinics in 350 existing health centres, but adolescence had not been recognized as a special sub-group (Albrecht, 1966).

In a leading article in the *Lancet* (1967) it was stated that the national child developmental study of 17,000 children born in one week in 1958 showed 10 per cent with emotional maladjustment by the age of 7 years. In another study quoted, of 9,200 adolescents tested, 6 per cent of these aged 10 to 11 years had definite psychiatric disorders, and a third of the total showed serious antisocial behaviour.

HISTORICAL REVIEW

As far back as 1860 psychiatric illness in adolescence had been recognized, for Morel (1860) described a case of dementia praecox in a boy of 14 years. Clouston (1891) wrote a paper on 'neuroses of development'. He considered 60 per cent made a recovery. Kraepelin (1896) defined adolescent psychosis, dividing it into manic-depressive, and dementia praecox. Burr (1905) discussed insanity at puberty. He divided cases into dementia praecox, original paranoia, mania, post-infective, sub-normal and hysterical.

Psychoanalysis came relatively recently to the study of adolescence (Masterson, 1967). It began with Freud's three essays on sexuality (Freud, 1953). Jones (1922) wrote an article on some problems of adolescence. Bernfield (1923) and Anna Freud (1927) were followed by Aichhorn (1935). Psychoanalytical aspects of adolescent psychiatry have been reviewed by Spiegel (1951) and by Anna Freud (1958).

In practical terms, however, there has been but slow recognition of the sub-speciality, although now a number of units have been established as specialized treatment centres to deal with the problem. Prior to this an artificial division between child psychiatry and adult psychiatry was drawn in the 15–16 year age range, cutting down the middle that group of patients where much of psychiatry makes its opening bow.

A special unit for adolescents was, however, set up at St. Ebba's Hospital, Epsom, as far back as 1949. The setting up of this unit is described by Annesley (1961). In the USA the first unit had been opened in 1937 at the Bellevue Psychopathic Hospital (Curran, 1939).

TERMINOLOGY AND DEFINITION

In reviewing the literature it becomes apparent that there are two difficulties which at once present in making valid comparisons. The first is that of terminology; the second the age at which adolescence is deemed, by various authors, to begin and end.

Thus, for example, prior to 1933, the term behaviour disorder was used loosely to describe phenomena that the child exhibited in dealing with himself or others that created difficulty in adjustment, e.g. enuresis, aggression, etc. (Wertz, 1962). Braceland (1937) however, defined a behaviour disorder as an undesirable character anomaly of a kind that renders the patient unresponsive to ordinary educative methods. Blau (1952) considered them to be special types of anxiety neurosis: 'Conduct disorders occurring suddenly in adolescence made one suspect psychosis, the real conduct disorders starting before $3\frac{1}{2}$ years of age'.

Some authors have attempted to delineate special diagnostic categories peculiar to adolescence. For example, Warren and Cameron (1950) discuss what they term reactive psychoses in adolescence. These were episodic and showed as a drop in scholastic efficiency with anxiety, sleep disorder, motor restlessness, disturbance of speech, perplexity, loss of contact with people, bizarre body sensations and occasionally hallucinations. They might be precipitated by physical or emotional trauma.

Similarly Masterson (1967) discusses the concept of 'adolescent turmoil', an adjustment reaction of adolescence used by various authors in their differential diagnoses of these groups.

Turning to the question of defining at what age adolescence begins and ends, we again find a variety of views. Henderson *et al.* (1967) in a survey of mental illness in Edinburgh described a group of patients falling between the ages of 14 and 19. Sukhereva and Kogan (1933) took an age limit of 14–17 years. Hall (1938) studied a thousand consecutive cases of 'juvenile nervous and mental instability', in an age group of 10–19 years. Warren (1965) included in his survey those between the ages of 11 and 19. Masterson and Washbourne (1966) took a group aged 12–18 years. Strictly speaking therefore none of these surveys are directly comparable, and this makes the problems of differential diagnosis more difficult.

A final problem is the question of defining a norm for adolescent behaviour, since many trials have been carried out without a control group.

The question of what is normal in adolescence in terms of psychological problems and psychiatric symptoms has, however, been discussed by Wilson (1960). Adolescents are considered to show episodes of anxiety, depression, hysterical symptoms, aggressive and delinquent behaviour, mild paranoid reactions, phobias and boredom! A leading article in the *British Medical Journal* (1960) also gives statistics about normal adolescents.

DIAGNOSTIC PATTERNS

Even when the above problems have been taken into account, difficulty remains in making accurate diagnoses, since the syndromes seen in adolescence are often ill defined, and are admixtures of symptoms found in more crystallized form in the adult.

Sands (1953) in his survey at St. Ebba's found that a third of those diagnosed were found subsequently to have been diagnosed incorrectly. Half could not be diagnosed at all.

Many writers have in fact tried to classify adolescent psychiatric illness. Thus, Kasanin and Kaufmann (1929) studied 160 patients under the age of 16 and found that 65 were psychotic, of which 21 were schizophrenic. They found that of these 21 only 6 were still diagnosed so at the end of the follow-up study.

Annesley (1961) in a study of 362 adolescents found 55 per cent behaviour disorder, 22 per cent schizophrenia, 9 per cent anxiety state, 8 per cent hysteria, 4 per cent affective and 2 per cent obsessional. McCulloch *et al.* (1966) in Edinburgh found in a group of 14–19-year-olds a referral rate of 9.08 per 1000. Of 373 referrals they diagnosed 7 per cent psychosis, 20 per cent neurosis, 26 per cent behaviour disorder, 12 per cent adolescent crisis, 11 per cent personality disorder, organic 4 per cent and in 11 per cent normality.

In another study in Edinburgh, Henderson *et al.* (1967) studied 230 patients, (106 male, 124 female). The diagnostic criteria showed that 9 per cent of the males were psychotic, 4 per cent of the females; 10 per cent of the males showed behaviour disorders, 7 per cent of the females; 17 per cent of the males showed personality disorders, 14 per cent of the females; 31 per cent of the males showed neurotic illness, 38 per cent of the females.

Masterson (1967) took a group of 107 patients aged 12–18; 41 per cent were diagnosed as acting-out problems, 25 per cent neurotic, 15 per cent psychotic and 9 per cent sub-normal. The sex ratio was two boys to one girl. Half the patients 'presented no diagnostic difficulty on initial interview' but in a few cases 'a definite diagnosis could not clearly be made even five years later'. Masterson studied a comparable control group of 101 adolescents. He found that anxiety, depression, and absence of a principal symptom pattern characterized 75 per cent of his control group and 37 per cent of the patients. On the other hand, schizophrenic and acting-out symptoms were present in 35 per cent of patients but only 9 per cent of controls.

Thus it is seen that not only are surveys not comparable for age, but the terminology used in deciding on diagnostic labels differs widely among various well-known authors. Often at follow-up they are shown in any case to have a wide margin of inaccuracy.

ASPECTS OF PSYCHOPATHOLOGY

Having thus far reviewed the scope and inherent difficulties encountered in the study of adolescent psychiatry, we will now turn to a review of the writings concerning the subject on which this book is essentially based, namely a consideration of certain aspects of the psychopathology of the syndromes seen in this age group, considering especially the questions of early environmental traumas, in particular separation experiences, and the development or otherwise of satisfactory interpersonal relationships. Finally, the identification of possible prognostic indicators must be considered.

Early writings on the subject largely consisted of surveys of diagnoses related in percentage terms to possible psychopathological events; thus Hall (1938) studied juvenile nervous and mental instability in 1000 cases between 1924 and 1937 using an age group of 10–19. There were 583 females and 417 males; 515 were conduct disorders, 448 had nervous symptoms, 37 were backward. There was a family history in 56 per cent of cases, I.Q. was of no significance, 45 per cent had had parental loss of one sort or another, 8 per cent were illegitimate, 14 per cent were only children. Prognosis was 29 per cent good, 34 per cent poor. At five year follow-up 40 per cent had made a complete recovery, 24 per cent a partial recovery, 17 per cent were unchanged and 19 per cent were worse.

Yearbury and Newell (1944) studied genetic and environmental factors in psychoses of adolescence. They took two groups of 56, patient and control; 42 of the 56 patients were schizophrenic. They found that hereditary tendencies were present in 38 of the patient group, 2 of the control; abnormality in siblings in 50 of the patient group, 2 of the control; bad home life in 43 of the patient group, 17 of the control; conflicting discipline in 33 of the patients and in 11 of the controls, brutal discipline in 22 of the patients and 4 of the controls. There was a marked lack of security in human relationships in the patient group.

These studies drew attention to the possible genetic factors involved. Similarly Schroeder (1939) took 51 cases aged 13–18 and found that second born were the commonest, there were few only children; 50 per cent came from broken homes or had had a dead parent, 7 were from foster homes.

Many studies have only considered prolonged separation. For example Caplan and Douglas (1969) defined separation as lasting at least six months during which time the child did not see the parent, taking an age range of six months to eight years. They showed that 50.7 per cent of depressed children and 23.2 per cent of those suffering from anxiety states had experienced such a deprivation and showed that early separation experiences were most common among depressed young people. Data from a normal sample were not obtained but they quote that in the general population in the USA 4.3 per cent of children had lost one parent by death by the age of 18, and 15 per cent were living apart from one or both of their natural parents.

A number of authors have attempted to compare developmental adjustment with subsequent breakdown, though usually on an uncontrolled basis.

Wittman and Huffman (1945) however made a comparative study of developmental adjustment and personality characteristics of psychotic, psychoneurotic, delinquent and normally adjusted teenage youths. The influence of broken homes was stressed in contributing to juvenile delinquency, more than 80 per cent of the adolescents in the control and psychotic groups had both parents whereas more than 40 per cent of the delinquents were from broken homes. A large number had been in foster homes previous to their admission to training schools. Of the delinquent girls 5 per cent were illegitimate. In considering parental relationships, the delinquent girls on average indicated that they loved their mothers much more than their fathers. The delinquent girl's father was described as of low average emotional stability, not affectionately demonstrative, a violent disciplinarian with no ambitions for the child's future. The psychotic patients rated their mothers as definitely below average in emotional stability, over-solicitous and over-protective. The type of adjustment made by the child with indifferent or rejecting parents appears to be of an overly compensatory sort, i.e. aggressive and antisocial. The child with the exact opposite type of parental relationship presents the picture of a severe personality disorder. The quantitative scores for home and school life indicated that family friction was definitely greater in the delinquent families than either the psychotic or control groups. They concluded that delinquent, psychotic, and control teenage subjects could be differentiated from each other in respect of sociological data, self-ratings of parental relationships, and early home and school life, as well as in personality type and adjustment levels. Personality type appeared to be of diagnostic significance only for specific diagnostic types among the psychotic group.

Warren (1949) in a Cambridge M.D. thesis entitled 'Abnormal Behaviour and Mental Breakdown in Adolescence', took a group of patients and attempted to assess aetiology, background and previous personality from the admissions to the Maudsley Hospital between 1945 and 1947. There was no control group. The age range of the survey was 14–18 years and he took 50 cases (24 female, 26 male). Warren found that there was no significant correlation with family history or serious physical disease. An examination of previous personality found a high proportion who had morbid traits dating back to childhood but no comparison was made with a normal group of adolescents. I.Q. showed no significance, nor did EEG recording. In factors emotionally ill-adapted to the patient in the family circle Warren considered (a) a bad maternal attitude, either rejecting, over-solicitous or nagging, (b) maternal absence, (c) paternal antagonism, (d) paternal absence, (e) material over-indulgence, (f) being an only child, and (g) major disturbance of home environment. He found there was a high incidence of maternal disturbed attitude in 80 per cent of the non-psychotic and 58 per cent of the psychotic group, 32 per cent of both groups showed maternal over-indulgence, 58 per cent of the non-psychotic group showed a major disturbance in home environment and 42 per cent of the psychotic group. Psychic trauma was found to be a precipitating factor in 30–40 per cent of non-psychotic and in 10–15 per cent of psychotic patients; over 50 per cent of neuroses began before puberty; 90 per cent of psychoses began after puberty.

Masterson *et al.* (1963) studied the psychopathology of adolescence with a control group. They studied 101 patients aged 12–18 years. Symptom categories were listed rather than diagnoses, with a principal symptom and others. It was found that these averaged 3 per patient. The five principal patterns were grouped as (i) thinking disorder syndrome, (ii) psychoneurotic syndrome, (iii) acting-out, i.e. the behavioural expression of emotional conflict, (iv) depression, (v) hysterical personality—the other 17 were not typical. Categories (ii) and (iii) were commoner in boys, (iv) and (v) commoner in girls, (iii) was commoner in the under 15 age group. They found that of the depressions 30 per cent had rejecting fathers, 83 per cent of the hysterics had rejecting fathers; 16 out of 17 of the acting-out group had rejecting mothers. Forty per cent had a history of psychiatric symptoms in childhood. Thinking disorder was related to early onset, and to family history but not to impaired parental relationships. Acting-out was related to early disturbed relationships with the mother.

Masterson and Washbourne (1966) showed in the same group that of the 101 healthy adolescents 27 had psychiatric symptoms of some kind or another, mild phobias or obsessions; in the patient group they found that family relationships were poor, there was a high proportion of absent fathers, there were fewer intact homes, the parents were often domineering, rejecting or over-solicitous and the adolescent was in chronic conflict with parents. The symptoms found in the normal group were anxiety symptoms, mild depression, obsessional symptoms, and very little acting-out. Of the patient group, 41 per cent had acting-out problems, 25 per cent had psychoneurotic difficulties, 15 per cent were psychotic and 9 per cent were retarded. The sex ratio was two boys to one girl. Masterson noted that the fathers of adolescents in the schizophrenia and personality disorder categories played an inadequate role because they were either absent from the home, disinterested in their child, psychiatrically ill themselves or excluded from the family by a domineering mother.

As regards diagnosis they found that approximately one half of the patients presented no diagnostic difficulty on the initial interview but in a few cases a definitive diagnosis could not be clearly made even in the five year follow-up study.

Masterson thus compared his patient group with a control group. He found that anxiety, depression and absence of a principal symptom pattern characterized 70 per cent of his control group and only 37 per cent of the patients. On the other hand, schizophrenic and acting-out symptoms are present in 33 per cent of the patients and only 9 per cent of the controls. Many more subjects in the control group had fathers who were present in the home. The relatively healthy had grown up in a benign atmosphere, tending uniformally to accept and to adopt constructive attitudes towards their adolescence. For the patient group family relationships could be characterized as poor, there were fewer intact homes, with a high proportion of absent fathers; psychopathology of the parent often manifested itself in his relationship with the adolescent through domineering, rejecting or over-solicitous attitudes.

Engel (1959) felt that in the neurotics the issue was a failure of the child to meet the mother's expectations. The non-schizophrenic sibling was more willing to disregard his mother's expectations than was his schizophrenic sibling. In the control group there was a better two-way communication.

Animal research has had an important part to play in considering the effects of deprivation experiences. Harlow (1961), for example, has studied the development of affectional patterns in infant monkeys. A most relevant finding is the intensity and persistence of the infant primate's monotropic attachment to its mother. Monkeys which had been separated from their mothers at birth and reared either in the absence of a mother surrogate or with only an inanimate cloth mother surrogate failed at maturity to show normal social and sexual behaviour. Despite this lack of sexual responsiveness four females were mated but it was noted that when their infants were born they showed a strikingly abnormal absence of maternal behaviour. This provides an incidence of a hidden effect of an early deprivation experience that only manifests itself in later life.

The sometimes long-term effects of brief periods of separation in infancy in rhesus monkeys has also been observed by Hinde and Spencer-Booth (1970). Five months after the separation experience, although their day-to-day behaviour lay within normal limits, the infants who had previously experienced separation approached strange objects less readily than did a controlled group.

Work with chimpanzees (Turner *et al.*, 1969) suggests that the social abnormalities resulting from separation experiences are modifiable only to a limited extent and then only with difficulty. Hinde and Spencer-Booth have shown that those monkeys which reacted most severely to separation were those that were already least well adjusted, and the same has been shown for children during hospital admission (Youle and Raynes, 1972).

We see therefore that a number of aspects of psychopathology have been studied and hints appear of possible important factors in the early environment being related to the occurrence of certain subsequent syndromes.

SUICIDE AND DELINQUENCY

There are two subjects which have been accredited special interest in the adolescent group and have received a large share of the literature. These may therefore be given brief separate mention in this review.

Balser and Masterson (1959) reported suicide as the fifth commonest cause of death in adolescents, being 2.5 per cent of all deaths in this group; 12 per cent of total suicide attempts are in the 15–19 age group and females exceed males by 10:1, the diagnosis of schizophrenia being high in the male group.

The *Lancet* (1964) discussed suicide attempts in adolescents and found that the ratio of non-fatal to fatal was 50:1, with a preponderance of females in the non-fatal group and males in the fatal group; 44 per cent of males proved to be schizophrenic. A study in Sweden found that only 4 per cent of attempted suicides had normal environments; most felt unwanted and often there was aggression against others and a hope of manipulating the environment and the attitudes of others by their suicidal attempt.

Teicher and Jacobs (1966) discussing suicide say that it is the fourth commonest cause of death in the USA in the 15–19 age group, surpassed only by accidents, cancer and homicide. They found excessive family conflict, broken homes, lack of meaningful social relationships and a history often of some insurmountable problem which caused the disintegration of any remaining close relationships and was the precipitating event. Sixty-six per cent of his group had a history of a previous attempt and 44 per cent knew of a friend who had made an attempt; 25 per cent had parents who had attempted suicide. One parent was missing in 88 per cent of cases; 42 per cent had step-parents, and in every case the adolescent was unwanted. Seventy per cent of the parents had married more than once; a quarter of the girls were pregnant.

Toolan (1962) discussed suicide and suicidal attempts in adolescence and found them to be common in the 15–19-year-old group, exceeding nephritis, leukaemia, tuberculosis and polio in frequency. Males were commoner than females in successful attempts, females were commoner than males in unsuccessful attempts.

Ten per cent of all suicide attempts occurred in adolescents. Of 37 in a series by Balser and Masterson (1959) 23 turned out to be schizophrenic. Ten per cent of adolescent admissions to the Bellevue Hospital had attempted suicide. There was a significantly higher incidence of first children in the family—49 out of 95 in one series—a higher number came from disorganized homes.

Considering parental separation of over three months as an aetiological factor, they found this to be present in the following:

(1) During the first year, absent father, 20 out of 95, absent mother, 2 out of 95, absent both, 7 out of 95.

(2) In the second year, absent father 9, absent mother, 4, absent both 6.

(3) Over second year, absent father 23, absent mother 2, absent both 11, out of 102 patients.

Delinquency has also been considered in the adolescent, since this problem has been identified as a problem basically of adolescence.

In 1951 an account of the psychiatric aspects of delinquency was prepared by Bovet (1951) for the World Health Organization—this remains a lucid and universally admired statement of the state of psychiatric knowledge on the subject. Cohen (1956) suggests that the delinquent feels he has an inferior status to the wider community and meets others in a similar situation. The delinquent group restores its standing while at the same time denying the values of the wider community. Hewitt and Jenkins (1946) distinguished syndromes which they called (a) unsocialized aggressive behaviour, i.e. cruelty, fighting, defiance and inadequate guilt feelings, which tended to merge with a factor of family parental rejection; (b) socialized delinquent behaviour pattern, i.e. stealing in groups, truancy, and running away, which occurred with parental negligence; (c) over-inhibited behaviour, such as shyness and apathy, which occurred in a repressive family situation. Destruction on a large scale is usually an indication of serious unhappiness and resentment sometimes displaced from the parents to the outside world. The background of parental rejection in its various forms described by Hewitt and Jenkins, is seen increasingly to produce not only severe emotional disorder but a delinquent prone personality, and the possibility of detecting children who are in special danger is being explored in child guidance clinics.

Bowlby (1946) states that for some years past half those people found guilty of criminal offences in the courts have been under the age of 21, and over a sixth of the total have been under 14 years. Indeed, of all age groups in the population it is the 13-year-olds who appear most often in court; thus theft like rheumatic fever is a disease of childhood and adolescence and as in rheumatic fever attacks in later life are frequently in the nature of recurrences. In order to assess the relevance of psychiatric findings in 44 thieves Bowlby compared them with other children seen at the London Child Guidance Clinic. These children were an unselected series of cases who did not steal and whose age and intelligence fell between the upper and lower limits of the delinquent group. Fourteen of the 44 were distinguished from the remainder by their remarkable lack of affection or warmth of feeling for anyone. They were conspicuously solitary, undemonstrative and unresponsive. The majority of these were found to have suffered complete emotional loss of their mother or mother surrogate during infancy or early childhood. Eighteen cases were found to have a parent or grandparent mentally ill. Only 5 per cent of the control group had had early or prolonged separation from their mothers. Bowlby included no case where the break was believed to have been less than six months. Pathogenic breaks appeared to have occured after the age of six months and in the majority after twelve months. Of the 27 children 17 had mothers who were neurotic and unbalanced in their attitude towards their children; of these, five stated that the delinquent child had always been unwanted and a sixth that she resented it being of the wrong sex. Separation to the child is often considered to be a punishment as a result of his own misdoings—a nagging, criticizing mother is not likely to make matters better and in some cases may clearly make them worse. Once the idea has developed, the child's guilt increases and a reaction of aggressive boastfulness may arise as compensation. The incidence of possible genetic factors was high both for the depressed and the hyperthymic groups of patients; the incidence of prolonged separation was far higher in the case of affectionless characters, i.e. 12 out of 14, than in any of the other groups studied; the incidence of hostile and ambivalent mothers was high in both the depressed and hyperthymic groups.

Summarizing, in the case of the depressed and circular thieves two factors are of principal importance, ambivalent mothers and recent trauma. In the case of the hyperthymics ambivalent mothers continue to be important, while other factors though present are relatively infrequent. Finally, in the case of the affectionless characters prolonged separations are of outstanding importance and all other factors are also-rans. Prolonged separations, as might have been expected from what has gone before, proved to be far more frequent in the case of the habitual offenders than in either of the other groups. Bowlby discusses the psychopathology of the affectionless character in some detail. He considers there has been a massive inhibition of object love combined with excessive and relatively uninhibited libidinal and aggressive impulses. This combination is clearly no accident. Thus misconceptions regarding both the motives of others and of their own 'unloveworthiness' develop, and in each case the resultant fantasy is common to all neurotics. If we are indifferent to others or dislike them we disarm them of any power to hurt us. This indifference was absolutely characteristic of every one of these children though in some cases it was little more than skin deep. It is a policy of self-protection against the slings and arrows of their own turbulant feelings.

Summarizing these aspects of psychopathology, we find that:

(1) Diagnoses fall largely into (*a*) personality problems in general (about 40 per cent), (*b*) neurosis (25 per cent), (*c*) psychosis (15 per cent), and (*d*) sub-normality (10 per cent). Approximately 6 per cent have a family history. Hereditary tendencies particularly are strong in schizophrenia.

(2) Suicide is the fourth commonest cause of death, and 10 per cent of all suicides occur in adolescence.

(3) Half the total criminal offences tried in court are committed by adolescents.

(4) With regard to childhood environment, in various studies 50–80 per cent have a disturbed early home environment, compared with 30 per cent of controls; 45 per cent have parental loss in childhood.

(5) Disciplinary habits are different in patient and control groups.

(6) Security in human relationships is poorer in the patient group.

(7) Rejection by or absence of father figures occurs in 30–80 per cent of some sub-groups.

SEPARATION EXPERIENCES AND DEPRIVATION

It is necessary now to turn to a more detailed consideration of separation experiences in those previous studies that have investigated this problem. It would appear that there is some evidence that there are critical periods of development in the child similar to that found in animal studies on imprinting patterns of behaviour. Deprivation, through separation from the mother figure, may disrupt patterns of development and emotional relationships which are forming at this point of time, and thus prevent imprinting from occurring.

Spitz and Wolf (1946) statistically analysed and supported with filmed evidence some groups of children and showed that the crucial period for the establishment of true object relationships occurred in the second half of the first six months of a child's life. During the first few months the child lives with his mother in a pre-object relationship which is based only on his needs and the anonymous satisfaction he receives. The smile at the sight of the mother's face is the first trace of a true relationship between mother and child and it is observed from the third month onwards. Towards the ninth month the child is capable of recognizing his mother without needing her. Spitz observed during this period real manifestations of anxiety when the mother disappeared.

Ethologists, for example Hebb (1949) and Erikson (1959), have shown that the process of maturation in many species may be arrested, and later stimulation of this process be ineffective, if severe stress or deprivation has occurred at a critical stage in the development of the young.

Corner (1944) states: 'Abnormalities are produced by attacking at just the right time a region in which profound growth activity is under way. Injuries inflicted early will in general produce widespread disturbance of growth, later injuries will tend on the other hand to produce local defects. If the child suffers sufficient pain through making relationships and having them interrupted that he is reluctant ever again to give his heart to anyone for fear of it being broken, his relationships with people from then on will tend to be under considerable strain. His desire for love, repressed though it is, persists and often results in behaviour such as promiscuity and the stealing of other people's possessions. Feelings of revenge may also smoulder on, leading to other antisocial acts.'

Many observations have been made concerning the effects of separation experiences and these can be conveniently divided into the immediate effects, the early after-effects, and the possible long-term effects.

Considering the immediate effects first of all:

Schaffer (1958) found that infants separated under the age of six months showed a global syndrome characterized by inactive, quiet preoccupation with the environment, a scanning of surroundings without particular focus and a lack of responsiveness to social advances. This varied in duration on return to the parents from 20 minutes to three or four days.

Bowlby (1951) states that all children under about 7 years of age seem to be vulnerable and some of the effects are clearly discernible within the first few weeks of life. Bakwin, (1942 and 1949) and Ribble (1943) have each given detailed accounts of the adverse effects on physical health. Bakwin, who gives a valuable survey of the paediatric literature on the subject which goes back to 1909, summarizes his own observations thus: 'Infants under six months of age who have been in an institution for some time present a well-defined picture. The outstanding features are listlessness, emaciation and pallor, relative immobility, quietness, unresponsiveness to stimuli such as smile, indifferent appetite, failure to gain weight properly, and an appearance of unhappiness.' These changes, he remarks, are not observable in the first two to four weeks of life but can be seen any time thereafter. The failure of such babies to smile at the sight of a human face has been confirmed experimentally by Spitz and Wolf (1946) while Gesell and Amatruda (1947) have noted a diminished interest and reactivity to be characteristic as early as 8–12 weeks.

Spitz and Wolf named this clinical picture as seen in the age range of 6–12 months as anaclitic depression. These very adverse results can be partially avoided during the first year of life by the children being mothered by an adequate substitute, although Ribble has expressed doubts that the reversibility can be anything more than partial and that damage is frequently done by changes even as early as the first three months. The nature of the response of the child to separation however may be misleading since often during the separation they are quiet, obedient and easy to manage. So long as they remain in the institution there is no obvious ground for concern, yet when they leave they go to pieces. It is evident that their adjustment had a hollow quality and was not based on a real growth of personality.

Goldfarb (1943) made a detailed study of this problem in children of about 3 years of age. On their return to their mother, for many weeks or months they may never allow their mother out of sight and they regress to babyish habits. Bowlby has observed acute phobic responses in children who have apparently recovered emotional equilibrium, when confronted by someone whom they associate with the separation experience. If the regressive anxious behaviour on return home is unsympathetically handled vicious circles in the child's relationship to his mother develop, bad behaviour being met by rebuffs and punishments, rebuffs and punishments calling forth more babyishness, more demands and more tempers. In this way develops the unstable neurotic personality.

Jackson *et al.* (1952) followed children aged 3–8 years through a tonsillectomy experience. On their return home, they reported that the common initial response to reunion was babyish and clinging behaviour with sleep disturbance, but after three months 16 per cent were still disturbed.

Pickerill and Pickerill (1947) suggest that regular visiting by the parents should be encouraged. Children between the ages of 3 and 6 years need frequent visiting, daily if possible. Older children can manage longer intervals. It is better to encourage mothers to drop in frequently and casually, perhaps when they are out shopping, and stay for brief periods during which they can feed and bath their children and give them small presents.

Burlingham and Freud (1942) write that the tears renewed at each visit are always distressing to the grown-ups who constantly feel that the child is best sheltered from these upsetting events. Only insightful understanding of the part they play in his future emotional development will enable the grown-ups to realize that they are worthwhile; an understanding made easier by recalling the value to adults of being able to weep over a bereavement.

Isaacs (1948) found that parents' visits were not detrimental to satisfactory foster home adjustment and, indeed, that the reverse seemed to be the case. Even before this, Cowan and Stout (1939) had carried out a systematic study in which they compared the degree of security shown in the behaviour of children who were permitted some contacts with their previous homes, with that of those who were not. Their results, using the records kept by the social workers responsible for visiting their homes, showed a statistically significant result, namely that 46 per cent of those who had contact with previous homes were insecure and 54 per cent were secure, whereas, in those who had no contact with their previous home environment 67 per cent were insecure and only 33 per cent were secure.

The League of Nations report (1938) laid it down that: 'It may, therefore, be regarded as an axiomatic principle of child care that no child should be removed from the care of an otherwise competent parent when the granting of material aid would make such removal unnecessary.'

The question naturally arises as to how long these bad effects from childhood experiences of this type may last. Is their effect permanent or not?

Mary Ainsworth, (1962) discussing the question of permanence of the effects of deprivation suggests that some damage is more obvious and more easily observable than other damage, and that it is very likely that some lasting effects are manifested overtly only under special circumstances later in life which reactivate pathological processes originally set in train by the early deprivation experience.

Even in gross measurements, such as I.Q., however, it appears that abnormalities may be found.

Goldfarb (1943) in a thorough study of 30 children aged 34 to 35 months, half of whom had lived in an institution and the other half in foster homes from four months of age, found a difference of 28 points of I.Q. on the Stanford Binet test between the two groups. The I.Q.s of the foster home group averaged 96, those of the institution children 68.

Other factors of a more subtle kind concerning character development may appear moreover.

During the late 1930s and early 1940s at least six independent workers were struck by the frequency with which children who committed numerous delinquencies seemed to have no feelings for anyone and were difficult to treat, and were often found to have grossly disturbed relationships with their mothers in their early years. In addition to Levy's paper (1937), papers were published in the USA by Powdermaker *et al.* (1937), Lowrey (1940), Bender (1947), and Goldfarb (1943), and in Britain by Bowlby (1940 and 1946). With monotonous regularity each put his finger on the child's inability to make relationships as being the central feature from which all the other disturbances sprang, and on the history of institutionalization, or the child being shifted about from one foster mother to another, as being its cause.

Meierhofer (1950) reporting on experiences with refugee children at the Pestalozzi village at Tholbert, Switzerland, says 'No doubt remains that a long period without individual attention and personal relationships leads to mental atrophy, it slows down or arrests the development of the emotional life and thus in turn inhibits normal intellectual development. We have observed that acute psychical traumas however serious do not result in such deep injury as chronic deficiencies and prolonged spiritual solitude.'

Most of the evidence in respect of long-term effects refers to the grave disturbance following severe deprivation. It is easiest to work from these established connections to those which are less well understood. The evidence suggests that three somewhat different experiences can each produce the affectionless and psychopathic character.

(1) Lack of any opportunity for forming an attachment to a mother figure during the first three years.

(2) Deprivation for a limited period, at least three months and probably more, during the first three of four years of life (Bowlby, 1951; Spitz and Wolf, 1946).

(3) Changes from one mother figure to another during the same period (Levy, 1937 and others). Certainly it would appear that the more complete the deprivation in the early years the more isolated and asocial the child, whereas the more the deprivation is interspersed with satisfaction the more ambivalent and antisocial he becomes. Bowlby asserts that if further research is to be fruitful it must pay minute attention not only to the ages and periods of deprivation but also to the quality of the child's relation to his mother before deprivation, his experiences with mother substitutes if any during separation, and the reception he gets from his mother when at last he becomes settled again. Bowlby noted that the separations which appeared pathogenic had all occurred after the age of six months and before the age of eighteen months; however, Goldfarb, examining social adjustment in adolescence in relation to the age at which they were admitted to the institution, points to the special vulnerability of the child during the first year in comparison to later ones.

Howells and Layng (1955) considering mother–child separation found no appreciable differences between their groups except for separations of over three months' duration. This occurred in only one of the control group but in six of their clinic cases. However, their follow-up time was not long enough to ensure that the later effects of deprivation could be identified.

Bowlby *et al.* (1956) discussed the effects of mother–child separation and did a follow-up study. He found a higher percentage of delinquents than normals had suffered prolonged separation in childhood. There were a number who were unable to make any mentally satisfying love relationship with other people and this group had nearly all been separated for over six months in early childhood. A much smaller percentage of the other delinquents had had this experience. There were marked differences between a group of foster children institutionally reared in the first few years and a group reared in foster homes from the beginning. He comments that in any one study it is impossible to isolate the effects of separation from the effects of other experiences. A group of children separated, because of tuberculosis, in a sanatorium were compared with a control group of their class-mates. More of the sanatorium children compared with the controls were unable to respond satisfactorily to a test situation. More were given to day-dreaming and lacked concentration; more were given to roughness and hostility. However, it was only a minority of the sanatorium group who were affected in this way, even though the numbers were significantly greater than in the control group. Further studies, with control groups, have shown similar findings.

An extensive study undertaken by Menut (1943) may be quoted. He compared 839 children suffering from behaviour disorders with 7000 control children from Paris schools and found that of the problem children 66 per cent came from broken homes while of the controls only 12 per cent did so. In a subsequent more detailed study he considered that in 84 out of 100 problem children the broken home had been the main causative factor.

Naess, (1959) however, who matched delinquent with non-delinquent brothers found that separation had occurred more among the non-delinquent than the delinquent.

Similarly Pitts *et al.* (1965) examined 748 patients with controls from admissions to wards of the same hospital. They found that there was no difference in terms of parental deprivation, between their two groups.

Lewis, (1954) found no special connection between separation from the mother in early childhood and any particular variety of disturbed behaviour.

These findings however seem to be in contrast with the majority of other studies.

Gregory (1958) reviewed possible sources of error in studies of parental deprivation. He found parental deprivation to be significantly higher in a delinquent group, early separation being more significant than later. Classifying by diagnosis he found an increased frequency of deprivation in psychoneurosis and schizophrenia, particularly occurring in the years under 7; it applied to both parents.

Differing techniques may be used to study the effects of psychological trauma on later adjustments.

Retrospective follow-up studies have included those of Lowrey (1940), Goldfarb (1943), and Beres and Obers (1950) who offer dramatic evidence in support of the hypothesis that early prolonged and severe deprivation of maternal care is significantly pathogenic. Bowlby *et al.* (1956) in a study of 60 children who had been admitted to a sanatorium for tuberculosis patients during their first four years of life and had stayed for varying lengths of time found that nearly two thirds were maladjusted enough to justify referral to a child guidance clinic. The patterns of difficulty in interpersonal relations ranged from marked over-dependence to clearly affectionless character formations. Stott (1956) also studied this subject. Stott's and Bowlby's studies do not throw direct light on reversibility but it may be inferred that since Bowlby's sanatorium children had normal intelligence and both samples included a number of seemingly well-adjusted children that there had been substantial improvement of functioning in at least some cases. The incidence and the severity of the disturbance, however, represented in Beres and Obers' sample suggests that any reversal of impairment that had taken place fell far short of completeness.

Robertson (1953) reported that all the children in his study who had suffered prolonged depriving experiences shared a common impairment—namely, an inability to form and maintain close and mutually satisfying interpersonal ties, although the manifestation of this impairment differed from child to child.

Trasler (1960) dealt entirely with separated children in foster homes, comparing a group of children unsuccessfully placed with a group that had been successfully placed. Prolonged institutional care during the earliest years of life, occurring after separation from the parents, and before placement with foster parents, was the antecedent condition most significantly associated with subsequent failure in the foster home, with affectionless detachment or isolation, rejection feelings and consequent aggression.

Donelli *et al.* (1965) studied the effect of maternal deprivation in Milan. They stressed the importance of a substitute mother in these situations. In a group of 123 patients, they showed that there was a lack of maternal care in 7.5 per cent, paternal care in 16 per cent, parental care, i.e. both, in 46 per cent, ambivalence in 16 per cent and deprivation of education in 14 per cent. These patients had a diagnostic category of character disorder (46 per cent, neurosis (35 per cent), psychosis (14 per cent), pre-psychosis (2.5 per cent), and epilepsy (2.5 per cent). They took as their age group however between 6- and 18-year-olds. They emphasized the importance of the first three years of life.

Another method of study has been that of *population surveys*.

Ainsworth and Bowlby (1954) stated with respect to the population surveys method that although perhaps attractive at first sight, an examination showed such a product to be fraught with great difficulty. The collection of the data presents the same problems as are met in the follow-up approach, multiplied many times because of the larger scope of the project. Douglas and Blomfield

(1958) studied 4668 children through interviews conducted by local authority health visitors with a pre-determined questionnaire. Through these interviews it was found that half the children had been separated at some time during the first six years of life although in only 14 per cent had separation lasted for over four weeks. This latter group was matched with non-separated children from the same population pool—the measures of emotional disturbance were crude and were based on answers to the questionnaire in regard to character disturbance, and no significant difference between the two groups was found, except when separations from both mother and home were considered. A follow-up study has been published more recently (Douglas, 1964) which to some extent modifies this view.

To summarize this section therefore, it may be said that separation has been shown consistently to produce characteristic effects in a large number of affected children. This type of effect appears to depend on the age of the child, the type of separation experience, namely its severity and the type of intermediate care, and finally the previous security of relationships before the separation experience occurs.

In most of the children the immediate after-effects of a limited separation wear off in a matter of weeks—though not in all, and in institutionalized children the difficulties are much greater. However, there may well be hidden personality defects only manifested later in life when something occurs to resurrect the old insecurities. Most work done has been on fairly gross deprivation experiences.

THE RELATIONSHIP OF SUBSEQUENT ILLNESS TO DEPRIVATION EXPERIENCE

Turning now to the question of childhood emotional trauma (and in particular the question of maternal deprivation), in relation to subsequent illness, Bowlby (1951) in his monograph to the World Health Organization comments that he is a little astonished to find how lightly early separations had been treated by most workers in his field; Burt (1929), for example, placed these early separations among the minor factors in the origin of delinquency although his actual figures hardly warranted such a conclusion since he found that 23.5 per cent of boys and 36.5 per cent of the girls had suffered prolonged absence from their parents. This contrasted with figures of 1.5 per cent and 0.5 per cent respectively for the controls. Bowlby's thesis in general was concerned with the interrelation of the affectionless character, persistent delinquency, and prolonged separation of child from mother. A further investigation was that carried out by Glueck and Glueck (1934). Here the age of the child when the break in the family occurred has been given—out of 966 juvenile delinquents 429 had come from broken homes, in 40 per cent of the 429, i.e. 19 per cent of the total, the break had occurred before the child was 5 years. A similar analysis by Armstrong (1932) had given comparable results—of 660 run-away children 29 per cent had their homes broken before the age of 4 and a further 28 per cent between 4 and 6; of 30 incorrigibles 40 per cent had suffered broken homes before they were 4 and a further 20 per cent between the ages of 4 and 6 years. Powdermaker *et al.* (1937) also found that of 81 delinquent girls studied between the ages of 12 and 16 years, 40 per cent had come from broken homes. Ahnsjö (1941) found that of 1663 girls committed to institutions for delinquency in the years 1903–1937 only 75 per cent had been looked after by both parents at the time of their birth and that the homes of nearly half of the remainder were broken through divorce or the death of one or both parents at the time the child was admitted to the institution. Similar findings were made in the survey of children in hostels for difficult children who had been evacuated from the cities of Great Britain during the last war (Ministry of Health, 1944). Here over 400 children were studied between the ages of 6 and 14 years, the majority being in hostels on account of stealing, behaviour disorders or enuresis. In this study no less than 45 per cent came from broken homes. Of the remainder nearly 25 per cent came from homes where although the parents were living together conditions were bad including cruelty, immorality, mental instability, unhappy family relationships, neglect or rejection; only 30 per cent came from homes which were complete and reasonably happy.

The findings quoted so far have all referred to the problem of behaviour disorders and delinquency. However, similar findings emerge in other conditions. Thus, in the League of Nations study (1938) on prostitution, findings were that between 20 and 30 per cent had lost one parent through death or separation while they were still young; in addition the percentage brought up in institutions, by foster parents, or relatives, was 20 per cent or more.

Early parental loss has been shown to be not only associated with depression but also with sociopathic personality (Earle and Earle, 1961), schizophrenia (Barry, 1949), and other neuroses (Caplan and Douglas, 1969).

Similarly a study of neurosis in soldiers in the Second World War revealed the high incidence among them of broken homes. Thus,

McGregor (1944) in analysing the findings of 2228 consecutive patients admitted to a military hospital for neurosis found that 48 per cent formed a personality group having the traits of timidity, immaturity, dependence and frustration. They came from broken homes or homes where there had been emotional stress in early life and this group revealed marked evidence of love deprivation in childhood.

Evidence shows that in schizophrenia broken homes are a common and significant feature of the history. Pollock *et al.* (1939) found a 'broken home' in the history of 38 per cent of 175 patients suffering from schizophrenia, and Lidz and Lidz (1949) in studying 50 schizophrenics who had become psychotic before the age of 21 found a similar incidence of 40 per cent. These high figures for schizophrenics contrast with a figure of only 17 per cent for a group of 155 patients suffering from manic-depressive psychosis, which is about the same as that of the ordinary population.

Unfortunately, the majority of these studies lack adequate control groups. However, some evidence can be found that in the general population the incidence of broken homes is approximately 12 per cent. Menut, (1943) and Madow and Hardy, (1947) quote three different American sources which show the percentage to lie between 11 and 15 per cent. It is not always possible to decide in these cases whether the results are due to heredity or to environment. However, Bowlby in his World Health Organization monograph quotes a study by Barry (1949) which showed that while death of the mothers was frequent in cases suffering from psychosis in adolescence, death of the fathers was no more frequent than in the general population and he suggested that this made it likely that the environmental factor was more important.

CRITICAL AGE OF DEPRIVATION AND OTHER TRAUMAS

The question arises as to what age group is particularly prone to suffer ill-effects from a deprivation experience.

Goldfarb (1943) bases his views on the importance of deprivation in the first year of life on a study carried out with children aged 12 years and over who had been in an institution for varying periods of time during their first three years of life. He selected 15 pairs of children matched for age and sex, half of whom were socially well adjusted and the other half a severe problem. He demonstrated that the differences in these children's behaviour could not be accounted for by the heredity or by the attitude of parents or foster parents; on the other hand there was a significant difference between the groups in respect of age of admission to the institution, the mean age of the well-adjusted being 10.9 months and the badly adjusted 5.8 months. No conclusions regarding the first half year are possible from his study however, but the legitimate and very important conclusion appears to be that deprivation in the second half year of the child's life has more far reaching consequences than deprivation occurring later.

In a later study, Barry (1949) concluded that the critical period for separation from the mother was before the age of 8 years.

Two major patterns of behaviour emerge in follow-up studies of separated children, one of anxious over-dependence, and superficiality and affectionlessness as the other. The anxious, clinging response following reunion after relatively brief separation occurred on the one hand, and the detachment and failure to re-establish affectional relations after long and severe separations on the other. Follow-up studies of children after reunion suggest that the overt disturbances after brief separation tend to diminish fairly readily except in cases where the child–mother relation was originally distorted, and provided that subsequent separation does not reinforce the process activated by the separation in question. That the overt disturbance disappears, however, does not mean that the separation experiences had no lasting effect—on the contrary, increased sensitivity to separation anxiety is at least one hidden effect that is grossly observable when there is a new threat of separation. The overt disturbance after depriving separations is clearly severe and prolonged.

Capes *et al.* (1971) studied a group of 153 adolescent patients born between 1953 and 1954 in the Wessex region. These adolescents were studied over a four year period. The majority had shown maladjustment under the age of five years. They stated that the assessment and treatment of such children should start before the age of five and not at fourteen or fifteen when disturbed behaviour becomes more manifest. This can only be done by identifying children at risk at the pre-school level.

The National Survey of Health and Development, a long-term study of 5362 young people now aged 27, showed that by the age of 15, 11 per cent of the families had broken up, death causing 296 of the breaks, and divorce 244. Nearly half the children from broken families still lived with their mothers and only sixteen were in institutional care. High rates of illegitimacy were found among girls from families that broke up when they were under six years of age. There was an increase in court appearances for the boys in this group and an overall increase in enuresis.

Douglas *et al.* (1968) in a national sample of some 5000 children showed that by four and a half years of age a third of children had been separated from their mother for at least one week. They found a weak association between brief separations and delinquency.

Stacey *et al.* (1970) have shown that some of the individual variations in the effects of separation and deprivation can be accounted for in terms of what the children were like prior to the separation experience. Infants who show the greatest disturbance following separation are those who have shown the most tension in their relationship with their mother before separation. It may be that children who have experienced separation become sensitized so that later similar experiences are more traumatic. Rutter (1971) quotes authors who have shown that infants produced little distress in a strange environment with their mother but considerable distress when on their own or with a stranger. Infants of about one year old normally reacted adversely to strangers.

Rutter states that separations which occurred in children already at a social disadvantage due to family stress or discord were more disturbed than separations which occurred in a secure environment for reasons such as a holiday. It may well be, however, that separation is disturbing to some children and not to others for a variety of reasons, and to identify those which one might expect to become disturbed would be most useful. Much of the work referred to has occurred, however, in the investigation of delinquent behaviour and there are many other types of problem which could arise later which might not have been shown in the particular cases quoted.

Gibson (1969) points out that a distinction must be made between separation and permanently broken homes, though the literature tends to confuse the two categories. Gibson quotes studies which relate to populations recruited before the onset of delinquent behaviour and shows that the percentage of those becoming delinquent is greater when the break has occurred after the fifth birthday but these figures do not reach statistical significance.

Since most children in care are only identified after they have been separated from their families one can never be certain to what extent the subsequent maladjustment is a continuation of previous behaviour, a reaction to separation or a result of the quality of substitute care.

If the important aspect in separation experience is the presence of a person to whom the child has formed a bond then it is the bond formation rather than the specific mother–child bond that may be important, and it would be in the child's interest to encourage attachment to several people at the appropriate time in its formative years.

Caldwell (1964) states that research findings have failed to show any significant effects stemming from patterns of feeding, time of weaning and type of toilet training, and the consequences of different patterns of discipline appear slight (Becker, 1964). Rutter (1971) states that most youngsters experience some form of temporary separation from their parents during childhood, one in three children having been separated from their parents for at least a week before the age of four and a half years. Most turn out to be quite normal and the question is posed, not should separation be allowed, but rather what sort of separation leads to psychological disturbance. Moreover it is misleading to regard separation as only from the mother. For example, when children are admitted to hospital with a brother or sister, they may show less distress, and although the separation is probably the principal factor even in hospital admission the type of care during separation is also relevant. Temporary mental characteristics prior to separation have been shown to be important and similar findings have been found in subhuman primates (Hinde and Spencer-Booth, 1970).

Rutter in his series showed that children separated from both parents came from more disturbed home backgrounds than did children who had never experienced separation, and many had been separated due to being taken into care in the context of long standing family difficulties. The largest differences in antisocial behaviour were found to be associated with their marriage rating and not with separation experiences. Separation from one parent only carried no increase in the rate of antisocial behaviour. He concludes that there was no association between separation from one parent only and any type of psychiatric or behavioural disorder in children. This does not rule out, however, the possibility of latent disturbances which may become manifest in later adolescence. Some studies, for instance, have suggested that childhood bereavement causes an increase in depressive disorders in adult life (Hill and Price, 1967).

During the early 1940s a number of significant studies were undertaken in the area of the influence of early experiences upon later personality development. Burlingham and Freud (1942) studied the frequently disturbing effects of the separation of young children from their mothers arising from the dislocations occasioned by war events. The work of Spitz and Wolf (1946) documented the sweeping and at times apparently irreversible psychological consequences of an unhealthy nature arising from institutional placements with inadequate mother substitute care. Prugh *et al.* (1953) discussed the masked deprivation which may be found in infants and young children even when the home is apparently intact. The child may have a specific but distorted meaning for the parent, producing a relationship of distorted relatedness, or the parent may be so involved in his own concerns that he is unable to provide adequate emotional supplies or adequate parenting for the infant.

Pringle and Bossio (1960) in a study of institution children considered that age of separation seemed important since 9 of the severely maladjusted children had been separated before 12 months of age while 4 of the 5 stable children had been at least 2 years old before the first separation.

Earle and Earle (1961) found that in a group of 100 patients who had suffered mother–child separation for at least six months before the age of 6 years, these patients being at the time of the study, adult, showed a significantly higher prevalence of sociopathic personality disturbance and behaviour disorders than a control group of patients. Among the separated group the prevalence of sociopathic personality was 27 per cent; in the remainder it was 2.9 per cent.

Wooton (1962) suggests that although separation from the mother before the age of 5 was found to be a prognostically adverse feature nearly a third of the children who were separated from their mothers were in a satisfactory condition at the end of the follow-up period, i.e. from 2 to 3½ years after admission, and permanent separation before the age of 2 years had not been the prelude to a particularly unsatisfactory condition of the child at the end of the period. These results, of course, ignore the long-term effects which such a short follow-up period cannot hope to ascertain.

It seems reasonable to conclude from present evidence that deprivation during the first year of life affects language and abstract functioning, and therefore indirectly the I.Q. or Deficiency Quotient (D.Q.) more than does deprivation later on. Lack of continuity of relations has its chief effect on the capacity for affectional ties, especially in instances when separation from the mother is repeated. The findings that children who have apparently recovered from a separation experience are particularly vulnerable to subsequent threats of separation, and that there is an empirical association between childhood bereavement and adult depressive illness, suggests that early experience may set up processes which may remain covert for a long time, but when subsequently reactivated by some stressful experience cause a pathological reaction.

PATERNAL DEPRIVATION

Little attention has been paid in all these studies to the role of the father. That this is not without some importance is shown however by a few studies, two of which are quoted.

Barry (1949) found that loss of mother through death, either in the first five or in the second five years of life, was an antecedent occurrence significantly more frequent among mental hospital patients than in the general population. Loss of a father through death was also an antecedent significantly more frequent among mental hospital patients than in the general population, but here the important childhood period was from 5 to 10 years of age.

Mathis (1964) states that relations between the mother and the child have received considerable attention. On the role of the father, which has not been very much discussed, he talks of a syndrome of 'carrence d'autorité' which occurs in juvenile delinquents. Mathis' study concerned 39 adolescents chosen at random between 13 and 18 years of age who were at the Centre d'Observation de Strasbourg Nøeuhoff in 1960 and 1961, coming from Alsace. They noted that 15 fathers were characterized by feebleness and a complete absence of authority. They say that consistently the child was found to reject the father and that often there was a complicity of the mother with the child against the father and disagreement between the parents. Frequently the paternal role was taken by someone other than the real father. They state that in all these cases the father was not really the protector of the wife and children, he was on the contrary an insecure element due to his feebleness or aggressive attitudes.

OTHER AETIOLOGICAL FACTORS

Finally one must turn to works—relatively few in number—which have sought to study other possible aetiological factors besides deprivation and separation, in the causation of adolescent troubles.

Wardle (1961) studying cases in a child guidance clinic, investigated the association of three sets of antecedent conditions with the type of behaviour problems shown in the child; (*a*) homes broken by loss of one parent through death, divorce or separation, (*b*) other child separations of over six months, (*c*) one parent having come from a broken home. He found that conduct disorders, including stealing, occurred significantly more frequently among children from broken homes, among those in intact homes who had been separated from their mothers, and among those whose parent or parents had themselves come from broken homes. Neurotic disorders were found more frequently among children from intact homes and who had not suffered mother–child separation. No significant differences were found, however, between those children from broken homes who had been separated from their mothers and those who had not.

Lewis (1954) focused on pathogenic pre-separation experiences. She dealt with 500 children admitted to a reception centre. Lasting separation of the child from the mother before the age of 2 years was one of 7 features of early parent–child relations and was significantly related to the degree of maladjustment, the other features being lack of maternal affection, maternal over-indulgence, maternal mental illness, paternal neglect, paternal over-indulgence, and prolonged public care. Parental rejection seemed a significant antecedent to unsocialized aggression; neglect by parents tended to precede socialized delinquency, while a repressive regime seemed associated with later neurotic adjustment.

The prior nature of the mother–infant relationship appears to represent an additional variable in the determination of the infant's response to separation. In this connection Spitz and Wolf (1946) suggested that the infant who has in general a closer and more intensely satisfying relationship with his mother may suffer more immediate effects from separation and may find the substitute more difficult to accept than the infant who has received more limited gratification from his mother. The unique conflicts which the young child may be dealing with during the stage when emotional trauma occurs may also influence his immediate response, the type of resulting symptomatology, and the later personality development.

Finally it must be remembered that different cultures bring up their children in different ways and a comparison of differing cultures may bring out other facets of the problem not seen when studying a single cultural pattern.

Mead (1962) contributes an interesting chapter on the differing methods which various cultures have of bringing up children, and how deprivation and the diffusion of mother–child ties affects the personality of the adolescent. For example, under group nurturing it appeared that the mobility and flexibility of a child's personality was impaired, but there seemed to be security in a larger number of nurturing figures. Rearing in such a setting leads to fecundity.

The ill-effects of deprivation vary with its degree. Partial deprivation brings in its train acute anxiety, excessive need for love, powerful feelings of revenge and, arising from these last, guilt and depression. These emotions and drives are too great for the immature means of control and organization available to the young child. The consequent disturbance of psychic organization then leads to a variety of responses often repetitive and cumulative, the end products of which are symptoms of neurosis and instability of character.

A consideration of traumatic situations in early childhood must take into account the phase which the infant has reached when the crisis occurs. In broad outline, the following phases seem to be the most important:

(1) The phase during which the infant is in the course of establishing a relationship with a clearly identified person, usually his mother, which is normally achieved by five or six months of age.

(2) The phase during which he needs her as an ever present companion, which lasts from about six months to about three.

(3) The phase during which he is becoming able to maintain a relationship with her without her presence being permanently necessary. During the fourth and fifth years such a relationship can only be maintained in favourable circumstances and for a few days or weeks at a time. After 7 or 8 the relationship can be maintained for periods of a year or more though not without strain.

PROGNOSIS

Some authors have suggested that adolescent personality disorders and in particular the so-called adolescent crisis will in most cases make a spontaneous recovery. However, well-conducted controlled trials suggest that this is by no means so.

Gillespie and Lay (1936) say that in a series of untreated school children few of their problems cleared up spontaneously, and that the prognosis in untreated patients is bad.

Carter (1942) discusses prognostic factors in adolescent psychoses and gives a historical review of the subject. He took 78 cases between the ages of 14 and 18 years, all of these were psychotic and represented 70 per cent of the whole. They were classified by Dawson's (1935) classification into organic, confusional, and biogenetic. Eight were organic, 10 confusional, 22 manic-depressive, 60 schizophrenic; 46 per cent made a good recovery but only 14 of these were schizophrenic. This was in a three year follow-up. Thirty per cent showed a family history; 70 per cent had a poor previous personality.

This type of study however means little in terms of modern treatment techniques, and without separating diagnoses or at any rate symptom clusters in some way it is doubtful if the figures are helpful.

Masterson (1956) states that little is known about the prognosis of emotional illness occurring during adolescence. He obtained follow-up information with a span of 5 to 19 years on 153 adolescent patients between the ages of 12 and 18, hospitalized at the Payne-Whitney Psychiatric Clinic. The patients were divided into four outcome groups based on their present level of functioning. For the schizophrenic patients in each group a rank T-test was used to determine the relationship between the clinical factors used in prognosis and later adjustment. Sixty-seven per cent of the schizophrenic patients had a poor outcome. Of 38 personality disorders 10 had a good outcome, and in the neurotic group of 11 patients, 11 had a good outcome.

An important point is the question of the total adequate relationships of empathetic type which the adolescent is able to forge and maintain.

Phillips (1953) found that the ability to form and maintain friendships during adolescence was positively related to prognosis. He attempted to measure (*a*) the frequency of interpersonal interaction, (*b*) frequency of group interaction, (*c*) complexity of social relationships, and (*d*) degree of passivity in interpersonal relationships. He found that the schizophrenic violates various norms and therefore others turn away from him, and this encourages his further withdrawal from social contact.

Sullivan (1956) too hypothesized that schizophrenics who lacked a significant interpersonal relationship in adolescence, outside the family, would have a poor chance of social recovery.

Pitt (1964) observed that the less peer interaction there was between the patient and his group the longer the hospitalization tended to be. The adolescent schizophrenic because of passivity and over-self-involvement is unable to interact, and thus he fails to secure access to many of the opportunities the peer group affords for the learning of adult behaviour.

Masterson (1956) found that most of the personality disorders settled in their early 20s. Good prognostic indicators were their response to psychotherapy, an abnormal EEG, an age of under 16 years at onset, a good school adjustment and a rapid clearing of symptoms. Discussing schizophrenia he considers that good prognostic factors are onset over 15 years, affective features, good previous adjustment and rapid recovery. Bad prognostic factors were an onset under 14 years, hebephrenic type of pattern or simple type of pattern, symptoms present for over a year, a poor previous social adjustment and a shallow affect. Sex, family history and precipitating factors he considered to have no prognostic significance.

TREATMENT

Early discussions on this aspect of the problem are no longer valid due to the improvement in treatment methods available. The question of psychotherapy is however important, particularly in those patients with personality disorders. As has been pointed out many of this group come in the category of affectionless characters.

Because of the inability of these patients to make relationships the psychotherapist is robbed of his principal therapeutic tool.

This group, therefore, have been described as having a poor prognosis. The findings of Powdermaker *et al.* (1937) in this regard are clear. Working over a period of six years in a home for delinquent girls, therapy was given to a group of 80. Half were successes and half were failures; response to therapy was related neither to intelligence nor to heredity; its relationship to the girls' early family experience, however, was striking.

Aubry (1955) and her associates, however, gave to a few individual children, who had suffered extreme damage from early severe deprivation, intensive psychotherapy with strikingly hopeful results in some cases.

Can one predict at an early age which children will become problems and need care and treatment? The presence of deprivation would seem an obvious pointer. Apart from this little reference is found in the literature on this point.

Daily (1959) presenting follow-up studies of children seen at the Dallas Child Guidance Clinic discussed the school characteristics of male adolescents who later became schizophrenic. His results indicated that the school staff perception of the pre-schizophrenic boy was essentially one of general passivity towards others and towards the school environment, with lack of interest in girls, group activities and sports; he was more careless, more dependent, more irresponsible and more submissive. He was less well liked by his peers. The second diagnostic sign was the student's perception of a small failure as a major defeat. In most cases the school staff were aware of the beginning of character disorders in these children but only a small number of the pre-schizophrenic group were perceived by school personnel as emotionally sick.

Bowlby (1951) suggests that there are certain basic hypotheses which still need testing: (*i*) The grown-up's capacity for parenthood is dependent in high degree on the parental care which he received in his childhood, the corollary being that neglected children grow up to become neglectful parents. (*ii*) Basic studies are required on the different patterns of family life and association. (*iii*) Surveys are required in each community to determine the number of children suffering from deprivation and the nature and relative influence of each of the known factors. These should cover normal children in the community and long-term follow-up studies should be arranged.

Yarrow (1961) in a comprehensive review of the literature on maternal deprivation stressed many of the same points that have been made above; the desirability of identifying the basic variables and concepts that have been indiscriminately combined under the term maternal deprivation; the importance of the developmental stage at which deprivation occurs, the significance of the duration of the deprivation and the like. His chief emphasis, however, is upon the desirability of research to analyse the deprivation experience into its component parts such as sensory deprivation, social deprivation and emotional deprivation.

2

RESEARCH

In this book, we have set out to look at certain aspects of adolescent psychopathology and to test certain hypotheses which have been considered in the above historical review, and I now wish to present the results of some work carried out by the author.

Two groups of adolescents have been studied. The first consisted of 50 consecutive patients between the ages of 14 and 19 (which seemed the most logical and appropriate of the various definitions of adolescence) who passed through the units associated with the Department of Psychiatry at Newcastle upon Tyne. The second were an equal number of adolescents matched as far as possible for age and sex, but who had no psychiatric history and were obtained from the casualty and other departments of the hospital. These two groups were compared for aspects of their early history, personality and symptomatology. The patients were followed up over an average period of two years, in order to assess prognosis and the accuracy of the original formulation.

It is the author's contention that many patients have, for one reason or another, a dearth of satisfactory human relationships on which they can depend. It was therefore hypothesized that the patient group would have significantly fewer of these relationships than the control group, and furthermore that the more difficulty the patient had in developing these relationships—for whatever reason—the worse would be the prognosis. A corollary of this should be that a psychotherapeutic technique designed to give the patient this kind of relationship should improve the prognosis in proportion to its degree of success.

In addition it was intended to test the hypothesis that separation experiences would be commoner in the patient group than the control, and to analyse the type of separation experience as far as possible. It was suggested that these experiences and other types of emotionally traumatic experiences in childhood might be related to subsequent personality traits and symptom complexes.

It was hoped to be able to identify prognostic indicators which would be of value in clarifying diagnosis and designing lines of treatment to alleviate the problems which had arisen in the adolescent's life pattern.

The patient group consisted of 50 adolescents who were suffering from psychiatric illness. Organic brain damage or epilepsy excluded the patient from the study and only those patients who had mothers alive and willing to co-operate in the trial were accepted. In fact, only one patient was excluded because of non-co-operation by the mother, but 11 were excluded as having no mother available, because of death or loss of contact through divorce from the family.

It is appreciated that a result of this has been to exclude from the study some of the more severe types of parental deprivation problems, but so far as the statistical significance of the results is concerned, this would, if anything, cause the patient group to be less dissimilar to the control group. Thus any positive findings of differences should not by this procedure be invalidated. In any case the nature of the study demanded full information from the adolescent's mother concerning early life events, so that this exclusion was essential if all data were to be comparable.

The patient group on admission was interviewed by the author and information obtained concerning past history, previous personality and present illness through the medium of an interview questionnaire, so that the questions were to a large extent standardized. In addition the patient's mother was interviewed and data compiled concerning the patient's early history and progress.

The patient group was then followed up over a minimum period of two years, and at the end of this time a further questionnaire interview was held with the patient, concerning progress, prognosis, and present adjustment. Again the mother was interviewed and the patient's general practitioner (or hospital doctor if the patient had been re-admitted) was asked to fill in a short form dealing with progress. From these various sources of information data could be compiled concerning the patient's subsequent progress from first admission.

The control group, which was concerned only in the first part of the project, consisted of 50 adolescents matched as accurately as possible for age and sex, obtained at random from the casualty department of the Newcastle Royal Victoria Infirmary. The same conditions for acceptance to the trial applied, except that in this case a history of psychiatric treatment precluded acceptance. This group and their mothers were subjected to an identical questionnaire interview, as that of the patient group. The data obtained from these 100 individuals were itemized in such a way that they could be placed on to Holerith punch cards for convenience of sorting. From these cards information concerning the prevalence of various features in the early history and personality of the two groups could be compared. Features which appeared of particular interest in this study, and in the two year follow-up study, were subsequently placed on data tape, and a correlation matrix obtained using a program already available on the KDF 9 computer at Newcastle University, and in use by the department of psychiatry, for this type of project.

From this correlation matrix, where a significant correlation between two features occurred, items could be read off and conclusions drawn. These questionnaires and the subsequent item sheets are shown in appendices 1 and 2.

The original questionnaires covered a wide range of aspects of the adolescent's history. However, the data extracted for punch-card sorting concentrated on certain aspects with which this study was concerned and which are now enumerated.

INFORMATION FROM THE MOTHER

Early history

Particular interest was paid to the following:

(1) The family history.

(2) Any episodes of separation of child from parents, particularly during the first few years of life, and the effect of these episodes; by whom the child was looked after, and the effect of being reunited with the mother.

(3) Sibling order.

(4) Milestones and difficulties encountered with early training.

(5) Relationships between patient and parents in the formative years.

(6) Methods of punishment used, and the attitudes and consistencies of the mother.

(7) Effect of starting school.

(8) Effect of puberty.

(9) Any traumatic situations that may have arisen, emotional or physical (such as hospital admission) during the early years.

Recent parental attitudes to the adolescent

From these data a picture was built up of the total mother–patient relationships, and the problems encountered during personality growth.

INFORMATION FROM THE PATIENT

Early history and environment

Many questions were asked which were the same as those asked of the parents, partly to see whether the picture presented by the adolescent correlated with that presented by the parent. In addition special emphasis was placed on:

(1) Personal relationships with parents and friends. In particular the patient was asked if he/she could confide in the mother, father, siblings or other friends, and how many friends the patient had had at school—whether close or superficial etc.

(2) School and hobby activities.

(3) Sexual education and problems related to this.

(4) Experiences considered traumatic by the adolescent (which did not necessarily correspond to those considered traumatic by mother).

Present personality

Details were obtained of the patients' attitudes and interests, in particular to:

(1) Ambitions
(2) Fears and phobias
(3) Energy levels
(4) Ability to mix
(5) Optimism
(6) Moodiness
(7) Obsessional traits
(8) Day dreaming
(9) Responsibility
(10) Guilt Feelings
(11) Mixing
(12) Publicity
(13) Impetuosity
(14) Ability to empathize.

INFORMATION ABOUT THE PATIENT'S PRESENT SYMPTOMS AND ILLNESS

A standard case history was taken in the usual way and details of symptomatology, length of history, etc. recorded. A provisional diagnosis using accepted diagnostic criteria from the international classification was made. Finally, results of psychological testing were recorded when available. All patients had an estimation made of their I.Q.s by Raven's matrices or Wechsler Adult Intelligence Scale (W.A.I.S.), and personality testing was available on some of the group. The treatment the patient was receiving was noted.

TWO YEAR FOLLOW-UP STUDIES

The patients were followed up over a minimum 2 year (maximum 4 year) period, and then were submitted with their mothers and the local doctor, to a further questionnaire (Appendix 1).

Here an attempt was made to set an overall picture of the patient's progress since leaving our care, and to review the personality as it now presented, and to record any residual symptomatology.

Details were recorded of:

(1) Re-admissions
(2) Treatment since first admission
(3) Present situation
(4) Present total adequate relationships.

These data were also itemized and included in a second computer program.

The following items were extracted from all the sources and placed on punch cards concerning all 100 patients:

Items with only two variables (e.g. yes--no).

(1) Patient number
(2) Sex
(3) Whether changed from breast to bottle before weaning
(4) Effect of weaning (good, i.e. no difficulty—difficulty).
(5) Neurotic traits in childhood (yes—no)
(6) Affectionate child (yes—no)
(7) Mother attitude (good—bad) to patient
(8) Mother inconsistency of attitude
(9) Mother attitude to child waking at night
(10) Over-indulgence
(11) Effect of starting school (problem—no problem)
(12) Effect of puberty (problems—no problems)
(13) General peer relationships (satisfactory—poor)
(14) School (liked—disliked)
(15) Sports (liked—disliked)

(16) Phobias (present—absent) unspecified
(17) Ambition (present—not present)
(18) Ability to mix (good—bad)
(19) Energy (high—low)
(20) Fantasy life (rich—poor)
(21) Moodiness (marked—absent)
(22) Optimistic outlook (yes—no)
(23) Responsibility (enjoyed—not enjoyed)
(24) Tidiness (yes—no)
(25) Appetite (good—bad)
(26) Impulsiveness (yes—no)
(27) Ability to empathize (yes—no)
(28) Self-rating re personality adjustment (satisfactory—not)
(29) Symptomatology
(30) Aggression
(31) Retardation
(32) Indifference
(33) Obsessionality
(34) Ideas of reference
(35) Rapid mood swings
(36) Endogenous pattern mood changes
(37) Depression
(38) Anxiety
(39) Phobias
(40) Insight
(41) Physical symptoms
(42) Sleep pattern—initial insomnia
(43) Sleep pattern—early waking
(44) Family history of psychiatric disturbance
(45) Suicide attempt in patient
(46) Thought disorder
(47) Prognosis on discharge (good—bad)
(48) Absence of father in childhood
(49) More than one separation experience
(50) Sexual problems (present—absent) with type (homo, auto, hetero).

The Holerith punch-card sorter could take ten variables on any individual item. Some items lent themselves to this e.g. I.Q., and the I.Q. could be divided up into ten divisions therefore if one so wished. The following items were therefore given 10 variables as below.

(1) Age of onset of illness
(2) Age of separation experience

(3) Age of traumatic experience in general, e.g. hospitalization; severe physical illness; emotional trauma
(4) Duration of illness when first seen
(5) Length of stay in hospital
(6) I.Q. (1 = < 70; 2 = 71–80; etc.)
(7) Sibling order
(8) Age of weaning.

In addition ten subdivisions could be made to classify the diagnosis (into schizophrenia, adolescent personality disorder, depression etc.), and similarly the type of treatment administered, whether predominantly psychotherapeutic, drugs, and if so what general type, ECT and so on.

Separation experiences were subdivided into those where cover had been good while the mother was away, where reunion had or had not gone smoothly, and the length of the separation experience.

The types of inter-family relationships and the ability of the adolescent to confide in his parents, siblings or friends, were also subdivided according to the degree and extent of his relationships.

Finally, an attempt was made to categorize the type of punishment used and the consistency of the parents in this respect during the child's formative years.

In addition certain rating scales were devised in an attempt to form a quantitative measure of certain aspects of the adolescent's functioning. These scales were quite arbitrary and to some extent subjective. However, it is important to realize that many of the problems and symptoms complained of *are* subjective and not amenable to objective measurement (e.g. anxiety features) and that what one wants to know is what the patient feels, for this is what is important even if objectively there is no evidence for the symptom that is measurable.

An attempt was made to rate the mother in the light of the data collected into good or bad in terms of competence in child rearing. This scale means only as much as its constituent questions and may be criticized as superficial. If, however, it were to highlight differences between patient and control upbringing it would serve the function for which it was designed. Thus in the light of points raised by previous authors and mentioned in the historical survey, data were scored, (the higher the score the worse the mother) by allocating points to each question on the scale and converting this into divisions suitable for putting on to the punch cards and later on to data tape if they proved of value. These data included such items as:

(1) Mother's general attitude to the child
(2) Mother's consistency in handling the child
(3) 'Night attitude' of parents (e.g. was child left to cry)
(4) 'Deprivation' punishment (the child being left to cry)
(5) Corporal punishment
(6) Conscientiousness of mother
(7) Over-indulgence of child.

The idea here is based on the belief that it is not one single factor in a child's upbringing, or one single experience, which carries much weight. It is the accumulation of situations designed to create insecurity that subsequently takes its toll. A quantitative measure of this kind may therefore bring out circumstances not seen when one aspect is considered alone.

A rating scale was similarly produced relating to the patient's total personality, on the basis of the answers to questions in the questionnaire interview. This might be called a 'personality maturity' rating.

A rating scale was made of the parents' opinions of the child's stability as a child, using similar criteria and including items such as:

(1) Affection
(2) Friendliness with others
(3) Neuroses in childhood
(4) Traumatic incidents in childhood
(5) Pubertal problems
(6) Problems when starting school.

A scale was devised of the patient's opinion of himself.

An attempt was made to rate the patient's 'total adequate relationships', that is to say the number and quality of the individuals in whom the adolescent felt he or she could confide if in trouble, and who would not let him down, as follows:

(1) Total number of close friends
(2) Confides in mother
(3) Confides in father
(4) Confides in siblings or close friends.

Finally an attempt was made to devise a rating of what can best be called mutual understanding between parent and adolescent, based on answers in the questionnaire which showed that the patient and parent had or had not a fundamental disagreement on what the correct answer should be to the particular question involved. This included questions on:

(1) Traumatic episodes in childhood
(2) Ability to be friendly and empathize
(3) Problems over schooling
(4) Presence of neurotic traits.

The question here was did the parent know or trouble to find out about the child's problems, and did the child trouble to communicate these difficulties, if present, to the mother? It was hoped in the above way to quantify this aspect of the relationship from simple questionnaire answers. If a child and parent disagreed the question was scored. If both agreed the score for that question was nil. Thus the higher the total score the worse the relationship.

At the end of the two year follow-up period further questions were asked concerning progress and the presence of residual problems. This aspect of the study formed a separate item sheet and was run through the computer to obtain correlations between the outcome data and aspects of the patient's early experiences and personality. The control group, suffering no illness, could not therefore be included in this program as the results would have been invalidated by the heavy weighting of negative answers in the correlation matrix.

To aid in quantifying the prognostic findings a scale was further devised entitled 'final adjustment rating' on the results of yes—no answers to the final questionnaire interview.

The first correlation matrix to be put through the computer was composed of questions picked out to try to show a relationship between the presence of illness in the adolescent (and its absence in the controls) and certain factors in the early history and personality, contrasting the 50 patients with the 50 controls. There were thus 100 individuals. Thirty-eight items were correlated, and some of these had up to 9 variables corresponding with the punch-card variables.

The following items were included in the first correlation matrix:

(1) Sex
(2) Patient/control classifier
(3) Diagnosis schizophrenia
(4) Diagnosis depressive
(5) Diagnosis anxiety
(6) Diagnosis personality disorder
(7) Age of onset
(8) Mood swing endogenous
(9) Suicide attempt
(10) Aggressive symptoms

(11) Obsessive symptoms
(12) Ideas of reference
(13) Anxiety symptoms
(14) Phobic symptoms
(15) Mood swings rapid
(16) Sibling order
(17) Family history (psychiatric)
(18) Childhood neurosis
(19) Parent rating/child rating ratio
(20) Mother competence rating
(21) Total adequate relationships rating
(22) Abnormal early history
(23) Patient rating scale
(24) Mutual understanding rating scale
(25) Presence of delusions
(26) Presence of mannerisms
(27) Relationship with father
(28) Presence of separation experience
(29) Presence of adequate mother surrogate
(30) Effect of separation
(31) Length of separation
(32) Separated at age < 6 months
(33) Separated between 6 months and 1 year
(34) Separated between 1 year and 18 months
(35) Separated between 18 months and 3 years
(36) Separated between 3 and 6 years
(37) Separated over the age of 6 years
(38) Prognostic assessment.

The second correlation matrix was concerned with the 50 patients at the end of a two year follow-up period. Twenty-three items were included in the data placed on tape. It attempted to relate outcome to the type of symptoms present, to the ability to form adequate relationships, and to the existence of early separation experiences.

The following items were included:

(1) I.Q.
(2) Presence of mood disorder (when first seen)
(3) Presence of obsessional symptoms (first seen)
(4) Presence of anxiety symptoms (first seen)
(5) Presence of phobic symptoms (first seen)
(6) Family history—psychiatric
(7) Childhood neuroses

(8) Unsatisfactory mothering (rating scale)
(9) Total adequate relationships (1) (rating scale)
(10) Abnormal early history
(11) Relationship therapy with transference relationship
(12) Patient followed up
(13) Residual symptoms
(14) Final prognosis
(15) Re-admissions
(16) Final patient view
(17) Final adequate relationships (2) (rating scale)
(18) Thought disorder (when first seen)
(19) Length of separation
(20) Adjusted age of separation—separated $<$ 18 months
(21) Separated 18 months–3 years
(22) Separated $>$ 3 years
(23) Final adjustment rating scale.

In this matrix symptom complexes were used instead of conventional diagnosis (cf. Masterson *et al.* 1963) to see whether this was more relevant than less reliable conventional diagnostic categories.

A further rating scale on 'total adequate relationships' was used at the two year follow-up, directly comparable with the first.

An attempt was made also to adjust the age of separation to take into account the I.Q. It was felt that the chronological age of separation might be less important than the mental age that the child had reached. Thus items 20–22 refer to the mental age of the patient and not chronological, this being worked out on the basis of the formula

$$\text{M.A.} = \frac{\text{I.Q.} \times \text{C.A.}}{100}$$

where M.A. = mental age at time of separation; I.Q. was as ascertained from psychological testing; C.A. = chronological age at time of separation.

Twenty-four patients were still under the occasional care of a psychiatrist, at the two year follow-up survey.

NOTE ON COMPOSITION OF CONTROL GROUP

The control group was matched for age and sex. It proved impracticable to match the group for further factors, such as socio-economic factors and I.Q. but since both groups were obtained at random from the same catchment area it was considered that the differences would not be marked. Since the control group was obtained from casualty and the patient group from in-patients, there is the possibility of bias, for example, in differences in personality (extroverts tend to go to casualty—introverts tend to be admitted possibly more commonly), and other factors. It is possible that casualty attenders would show a higher neurotic score but this latter should not affect differences detrimentally in the study, and at any event the nature of the study prevented these factors from being completely eliminated.

3

RESULTS AND DISCUSSION

These are described under the following headings:

I. General information:

(1) Sex

(2) Age of onset—length of stay

(3) Diagnoses

(4) Symptom clusters

(5) Family history

(6) Sibling order.

II. Studies concerning separation experiences.

III. Relationship of childhood traumatic experiences to personality and diagnosis.

IV. The concept of 'total adequate relationships' related to psychopathology.

V. The concept of 'relationship therapy' and its connection with total adequate relationships and prognosis.

VI. Prognostic indicators.

In each of the sections (which correspond generally to the hypotheses to be tested) the following pattern was adhered to.

In order to test for significance a X^2 value was obtained using the formula

$$X^2 = \frac{N((AD - BC) - N/2)^2}{(A + B)\ (C + D)\ (A + C)\ (B + D)}$$

where N = total number of individuals (100) and A, B, C, and D refer to the numbers and frequencies of the two items to be compared. Since both rows and columns have fixed totals the d.f.

(degrees of freedom) equals 1. From Fisher's table of X^2 the significance of a given result can be read off. In the above circumstances X^2 must be > 3.841 to be significant at the 0.05 level, and >6.635 to be significant at the 0.01 level. A figure of >2.706 would be significant at the 0.10 level. Yates correction for continuity ($N/2$) is included in the formula.

Finally in each section the results of the correlation matrices are presented as appropriate. A discussion of the results is included at the end of each section.

The full correlation matrices are to be found with their key in appendix 3, but, as many of the figures are not significant and not relevant to the particular point under study they are not given in full in the individual sections.

The first correlation matrix concerned itself with diagnosis, personality, and childhood traumatic experiences, in particular separation from the mother, and related the 50 patients to the 50 in the control group. There were thus 100 individuals in the matrix, with 38 items to correlate with each other.

To be significant at the 5 per cent level a figure of ≤ 0.2000 is required, at the 1 per cent level a figure of ≤ 0.2600, and at the 0.1 per cent level a figure of ≤ 0.3200.

The second matrix was concerned with the two year follow-up, and thus contained only 50 individuals, all patients, relating their symptomatology, total adequate relationships and childhood traumas (especially separation experiences) with treatment, follow-up and prognosis. It contained 23 items correlated one with another, and in this case to be significant at a 5 per cent level a figure of ≤ 0.2800 was required, for a 1 per cent level of significance a figure of ≤ 0.3600, and at the 0.1 per cent level, a figure of ≤ 0.4500.

The correlation technique used has been the product-moment method, since this was the technique in use at the department, and is more accurate than the simpler rank-difference correlation method, since it takes into account the absolute size of the measures and not merely rank order.

I. GENERAL INFORMATION

One hundred individuals were interviewed, 50 of whom were patients admitted to the units in Newcastle upon Tyne at which the author was working. Fifty were adolescents seen in the casualty departments, who had no psychiatric history, and acted as a control group.

(1) Sex

Table 1 shows the sex of the patients; 38 per cent were male, 62 per cent were female. This female preponderance may be due to the tendency for male personality disorders to be dealt with by the courts and females by the medical services.

Table 1

Sex of Patient and Control Groups

	Patient	*Control*
Male	19	16
Female	31	34
Total	50	50

There was no significant correlation between sex and diagnosis. A correlation at the 5 per cent level of significance was found with the rating of mutual trust between mother and adolescent (i.e. mothers knew their daughters better than their sons; correlation = 0.2233).

(2) Age of onset and length of stay

One patient, a schizophrenic, had shown symptoms by the age of 6 years, and four were showing symptoms by the age of 12 years (patients 1, 13, 18, 22 and 37). Of the rest, four appeared in the 13–14 year age group, 11 in the 15–16 year group, 9 in the 17–18 year group, and 11 over 18 years of age.

The length of stay of the patients varied considerably but this may relate to a number of factors not directly the result of the illness, e.g. interest shown in the case, and the environmental situation to which they were to return. Three stayed less than a week in the unit: a further seven stayed less than a month. Three stayed over six months (cases 1, 28 and 50). Of the remainder, 18 stayed 4–8 weeks and 19 between 8 weeks and 24 weeks.

(3) Diagnosis

The diagnoses fell into the following categories and in Table 2 is shown the relationship of first to final diagnosis.

Table 2

Diagnostic Groups Compared on First Admission—Follow-up

Diagnosis	*1st admission*	*Alteration*	*2 year follow-up*
Schizophrenia	10	4	8
Affective	7	6	2
Hysterical personality	6	3	4
Anxiety state	10	7	7
Reactive depression	7	2	8
Personality disorder	8	2	19
Obsessional state	2	0	2
Total	50	24	50

(4) Symptom clusters

If symptom clusters are considered instead of conventional diagnosis it is found that there are many patients who overlap and show symptoms that would normally fall into more than one diagnostic category (Masterson *et al.*, 1963).

This is shown in Table 3.

Thus it is seen that 50 per cent of the diagnoses had been revised at the end of the follow-up period, chiefly in the direction of a diagnosis of adolescent personality disorder.

Broken down it is found that two schizophrenics turned out to be personality disorders, one an affective illness and one an anxiety state. Those diagnosed initially as affective became schizophrenic in one case, personality disorders in two cases and anxiety states in three. Three hysterical personalities became adolescent personality disorders.

One anxiety state became an hysterical personality. Four anxiety

Table 3

Presence of Symptoms in Patient Group

Patient number	1	2	3	4	5	6	7	8	9	10	11	12	13	14	15	16	17	18	19	20	21	22	23	24	25	26	27	28	29	30	31	32	33	34	35	36	37	38	39	40	41	42	43	44	45	46	47	48	49	50
Phobias	−	+	+	−	−	−	+	+	+	+	−	+	+	+	+	−	+	−	+	+	+	+	−	+	−	+	+	−	−	+	−	−	+	−	−	+	+	+	−	−	+	+	−	−	−	+	−	+	+	+
Anxiety	+	+	−	+	−	−	+	+	+	−	−	+	−	+	+	+	−	−	+	+	+	+	+	+	−	+	−	+	−	+	+	−	+	−	−	−	+	−	+	+	+	−	+	+	+	−	−	+	+	−
Depersonalization	−	−	−	−	−	−	−	−	−	−	−	−	+	−	−	+	−	−	+	+	−	−	+	−	+	−	−	−	−	−	−	−	−	−	−	−	−	−	+	+	−	−	−	−	−	−	−	+	−	−
Depression	+	−	+	−	+	−	+	−	−	+	−	+	+	+	+	+	+	+	+	+	+	+	+	+	+	+	+	+	+	+	−	−	−	+	−	+	+	+	+	−	+	+	−	−	+	+	+	+	+	−
Retardation	−	−	−	−	−	−	−	+	−	+	−	−	−	−	−	−	−	−	−	+	−	−	+	−	+	−	−	+	−	+	−	+	−	−	−	−	−	−	−	−	−	−	−	−	−	+	+	−	−	+
Aggression	+	−	−	+	−	−	+	−	−	−	−	−	+	−	−	−	−	−	−	−	−	−	−	−	+	−	−	−	−	−	−	+	+	+	−	−	−	−	−	−	−	−	−	−	−	−	−	−	−	−
Moodiness	−	−	+	+	+	−	+	−	−	−	−	−	+	+	+	+	−	−	−	−	+	+	−	−	−	+	+	−	−	+	−	−	−	+	−	−	−	−	−	−	−	−	−	−	+	−	−	−	+	−
Thought disorder	+	−	−	+	+	+	+	+	−	+	−	+	−	−	+	−	−	−	+	+	−	−	−	−	−	−	−	+	+	−	−	+	−	−	+	−	−	+	−	−	−	−	+	−	−	−	+	−	−	+

states became personality disorders and two became reactive depressions.

Two reactive depressions became personality disorders.

One personality disorder turned out to be schizophrenic, one was later diagnosed as a reactive depression.

The conclusion here seems to be that diagnosis is unreliable! At the final count 20 per cent of the patients turned out to be psychotic, 30 per cent were personality disorders of one sort or another and 42 per cent neuroses. Endogenous depression was uncommon.

Twenty-nine of the patients showed phobic symptoms, as did twenty-seven of the control group, and in this phobias differed markedly from other symptoms and seemed to be irrelevant in terms of distinguishing psychiatric illness from normality.

Thirty patients expressed anxiety as a symptom. Thirty-six patients admitted to periods of depression, despite the dearth of depressive illness in the series.

Symptoms of thought disorder totalled eight with delusional ideation; ten showing ideas of reference and ten with incongruity of affect.

Retardation appeared in 11 patients; depersonalization phenomena in 9. Aggressiveness was found in 8, and moodiness in 16.

Symptom clusters showed certain correlations on the matrix with other items, which will be dealt with in full later but are here briefly summarized:

(*a*) Phobic symptoms correlated with good prognosis at a level of 0.3110, significant at the 5 per cent level, and with follow-up good 'total adequate relationships' at a 5 per cent level of 0.2935.

(*b*) Thought disorder showed a significant correlation with the following items:

(i) With family history, 1 per cent level + 0.3825
(ii) With re-admissions, 5 per cent level + 0.3013
(iii) With length of separation, 5 per cent level + 0.2813
(iv) With age of separation,
M.A. $<$ 18 months 3 per cent + 0.3425
M.A. $>$ 3 years 5 per cent + 0.2735

Standard diagnostic categories also showed many positive correlations which will be discussed later. They are here tabulated for convenience.

No other items showed a significant correlation with depressive illness, but the numbers were too small to expect this.

Table 4

Schizophrenia—Relevant Correlations

Item	*Correlation*	*Significance (per cent)*
Family history	+ 0.4135	0.1
Sibling order	—	
Childhood neurosis	—	
Inadequate mother relationship	+ 0.1400	*
Total adequate relationships	− 0.1935	†
Abnormal early history	+ 0.1536	*
Separation as a whole	+ 0.1528	*
Separation experiences with an inadequate mother surrogate	+ 0.4225	0.1
Separation experiences with problems following reunion	+ 0.2703	1
Length of separation	+ 0.2842	1
Separation experiences at age 3–6 years	+ 0.3160	0.1
Separation experience at age > 6 years	+ 0.3408	0.1
Bad prognosis	+ 0.4955	0.1

* not significant; † nearly significant

Table 5

Depression—Relevant Correlations

Item	*Correlation*	*Significance (per cent)*
Family history	—	
Separation age 3–6 years	+ 0.2633	1
Suicide attempt	—	
Total adequate relationships	—	
Abnormal early history	—	
Prognosis	—	

Table 6

Anxiety State—Relevant Correlations

Item	*Correlation*	*Significance (per cent)*
Family history	+ 0.2007	5
Childhood neurosis	+ 0.1613	n.s.
Unsatisfactory mother	—	
Total adequate relationships	—	
Abnormal early history	—	
Separation experiences	—	
Prognosis	—	

n.s. not significant

Table 7

Adolescent Personality Disorder—Relevant Correlations

Item	*Correlation*	*Significance (per cent)*
Sibling order	—	
Family history	—	
Childhood neurosis	+ 0.2188	5
Unsatisfactory mother	—	
Total adequate relationships	− 0.2751	1
Abnormal early history	+ 0.2242	3
Suicide attempt	+ 0.3862	0.1
Mother–adolescent relationship	− 0.3922	0.1
Father relationship	− 0.2602	1
Separation experience	+ 0.2208	3
Age of separation experience 18 months–3 years	+ 0.2254	3
Prognosis	—	

(5) Family history

An attempt was made to relate the presence of a positive family history of psychiatric disturbance in close relatives with aspects of the adolescents' functioning. Family history was related to diagnosis on the Holerith punch cards and this is shown in Table 8.

Table 8

Family History Related to Diagnosis

Diagnostic Category	*Positive Family History*	*Negative Family History*	*Total Number*
None	4	46	50
Schizophrenia	7	3	10
Depressive illness	2	5	7
Hysterical personality	5	1	6
Anxiety state	3	7	10
Depressive reaction	3	4	7
Personality disorder	2	6	8
Obsessional	0	2	2
Total	26	74	100

The numbers in individual diagnostic categories are not large enough to make a valid X^2 test but if this test is applied to a comparison of the patient and control groups as a whole, it is found that, taking patient/control against family history/no family history

Thus

	Family History	No Family History
	a	b
Patient	22	28
Control	4	46
	c	d

and following the formula for deriving X^2 as stated earlier, that $X^2 = 15.2$ and this is significant at well over the 0.01 level, i.e.

there is much less than a 1:100 chance of this figure being obtained by chance.

If the results of the correlation matrix are now taken into account as they relate to family history, the results are shown in Table 9. Here a correlation at the 0.1 per cent level is found between family history and adolescent breakdown and this is seen to be particularly significant in the schizophrenic group and less so in the others.

Table 9

Relevant Correlations Referable to Family History

Item	*Correlation*	*Significance (per cent)*
Patient/control	+ 0.4104	0.1
Schizophrenia	+ 0.4135	0.1
Depression	—	
Anxiety	+ 0.2007	5
Personality disorder	—	
Suicide attempt	—	
Phobias	—	
Childhood neurotic traits	+ 0.2739	1
Unsatisfactory mother	+ 0.2262	5
Separation experience	+ 0.2044	5
Separation at 3–6 years of age	+ 0.2280	5
Abnormal early history	+ 0.2097	5
Bad prognosis	+ 0.3895	0.1

(6) Sibling order

Some authors have considered that the position of the sibling in the family is of significance—the only child may be especially vulnerable—the middle child may be vulnerable. The first child who is an only child until the arrival of the next sibling may show particular problems. Sibling order was therefore analysed as it related to factors in the matrix.

Table 10 shows sibling order of the patient group as it relates to diagnosis.

Table 10

Sibling Order Related to Diagnostic Classification

	Diagnosis							
Sibling Order	*Schizophrenia*	*Endogenous Depression*	*Hysterical Personality*	*Anxiety State*	*Depressive Reaction*	*Adolescent Personality Disorder*	*Obsessional*	*Total*
Only child	1	0	0	3	3	3	1	11
First child	3	1	2	1	2	6	0	15
Second of two	0	1	0	1	1	4	0	7
Middle child	2	0	1	0	0	0	1	4
Last of three	0	0	1	0	0	2	0	3
Later children of large families	2	0	0	2	2	4	0	10
Total	8	2	4	7	8	19	2	50

The scatter here shows no special grouping and is even throughout the scattergram.

Table 11 shows the relationship between patient and control groups, with regard to sibling order.

The only point of interest here is that there are fewer middle children in the patient group (10 to 4) and a larger representation of children of large families in the patient group. A X^2 test on these two items shows for middle children a X^2 of 2.07, and for children of large families, $X^2 = 1.25$.

Table 11

Sibling Order Related to Patient/Control

Sibling Order	*Patient*	*Control*	*Total*
Only child	11	10	21
First child	15	13	28
Second of two	7	9	16
Middle child	4	10	14
Last of three	3	3	6
Later child of large family	10	5	15
Total	50	50	100

DISCUSSION

(1) Sex of patients

The pattern of admissions in Newcastle in this age group was generally a preponderance of female to male, about 3 female to 2 male. A possible reason for this is suggested. Henderson *et al.* (1967) found a ratio of 5 male to 6 female in Edinburgh, but these included all out-patients. Masterson (1967) found 2 male to 1 female but included delinquency in his survey. The differences would appear to be the results of differences in the composition of the groups studied.

(3) and (4) Diagnoses and symptomatology

The difficulties inherent in making comparisons between different studies in terms of diagnosis have been discussed. It will be noted that the follow-up diagnosis had been changed in nearly 50 per cent of cases at the end of the two years. Twenty per cent of the cases however, were psychotic (16 per cent schizophrenic). This compares generally with Masterson's (1967) survey which is probably the most comparable. Symptom clusters were studied also in Masterson's thesis (1967) in the USA. Thirty-seven per cent of his patients had no dominant symptom cluster. Psychotic features were present in 33 per cent but this included those showing 'acting-out' behaviour. In the present series 20 per cent showed thought disorder. Symptom clusters remained more reliable as a guide to prognosis. There was a significant correlation with family history and interestingly with the more severe separation experiences at what one might postulate as critical ages of development. Phobias and anxiety states did not show these features but the former were good pointers towards final outcome.

Dealing with conventional diagnostic categories (final diagnosis) schizophrenia, as might be expected, showed a strong family history. The 'total adequate relationships' (T.A.R.) index gave a negative correlation suggesting these patients were poor mixers and did not easily develop confiding relationships. There was no significant correlation with separation experiences as a whole (see Table 4). Separation at certain ages was significant—the longer the separation the stronger the correlation, and the more traumatic the separation the stronger the correlation. Similarly reunion produced more problems in this group. This does not necessarily argue cause and effect since potential schizophrenics might react less well to this kind of situation than normal children. Also the numbers in the group were small. However, in the light of some of the work by ethologists the suggestion of a critical period in which age of separation proved to have a significant correlation is certainly interesting.

The numbers in the depression group were too small to expect significant correlations. Again, however, the relationship with a certain age of separation is suggestive.

Anxiety states show no relevant correlations with separation experiences. A positive correlation with family history may imply an environmental aetiology as much as a genetic one.

The more interesting correlations were those of the larger group of adolescent personality disorders. This group showed poor relationships with family and friends, significant at the 1 per cent level when compared with controls. Most of those who made suicide attempts came in this group. There was a 5 per cent correlation with childhood neurosis and a highly significant negative correlation and therefore poor relationship with both parents. Separation experiences were common and in particular a separation between the ages of 18 months and 3 years, again suggestive that this might be a critical period in development. This diagnosis did not relate to poor prognosis.

(5) Family history

A family history was present in the majority of those patients finally diagnosed as schizophrenic. It also distinguished between patient and control groups with a high level of significance. It is interesting that those with a family history also tended to have unsatisfactory mothers, no doubt because of the disability suffered in part by the parent. Childhood neurotic traits were found more commonly where there was a family history, and interestingly separation experiences were common in those with a family history—possibly because parental ill-health contributed towards the need for a separation experience. These items, therefore, all seem interrelated, supporting the view that it is the total environment that must be quantitatively measured to show a relationship with adolescent breakdown. A bad prognosis was common in those with a family history, probably due to the high weighting of schizophrenics.

(6) Sibling order

Table 10 demonstrates that diagnosis does not relate to sibling order, at any rate in the numbers available in this study. Middle children were found less commonly in the patient group but this only at a level of $P = 0.1$. The correlation matrix shows an abnormal early history to occur more commonly in only children. There are many possible reasons for this. The presence of a large family may shield the sibling. Parents who have only one child may be people who in various ways have more problems than those who go in for a larger family. They may be less fertile, and so on. The only fact is that only children are apparently at higher risk.

II. SEPARATION EXPERIENCES

Separation experiences as here defined refer to episodes in the early years of a child's life when child and mother were apart for a period of more than 72 hours. Much has been written about severe deprivation and about prolonged separation experiences. In this study the separation experience as above defined has been investigated from the point of view of the age at which a separation experience occurred, the length of time that the separation experience lasted, the circumstances of the separation and what kind of substitute the child had during the experience as 'stand-in' for the mother, and finally the immediate after-effects of being reunited. These aspects of separation have then been compared between patient and control groups, and related to aspects of personality, and diagnostic formulation in the correlation matrix. The results of these investigations are now presented.

(1) Total numbers

Of the 50 patients under investigation, eighteen (36 per cent) had been subjected to a separation experience. Of these, ten had been of less than two weeks' duration, and eight had been more prolonged. The arrangements for 'cover' during separation had been poor in seven, and there had been marked difficulties in terms of the child's behaviour afterwards, in seven also, of which five were the same cases.

In the control group there were 8 (16 per cent) separation experiences, five of which were under two weeks' duration, and only three prolonged. Cover had been poor in two cases and difficulties had been experienced afterwards with these two and with a third where cover had been apparently adequate.

Subjecting these total figures to a X^2 test, it is found that X^2 for separation related to patient/control equals 4.22 which is significant at the 0.05 level. The correlation is 0.2478 which is just under the 1 per cent level of significance.

(2) Age of separation

The age at which separation experiences occurred was broken down by punch-card sorting and the results shown in Table 12.

It is found using the results of the correlation matrix that there is a positive correlation of 0.2676 (i.e. 1 per cent significance level) between the patient group and separation between the ages of 18 months and 3 years.

Table 12

Age of Separation Related to Patient/Control Groups

Age of Separation	*Patient*	*Control*
None	32	42
< 6 months	4	0
6 months–1 year	1	4
1 year–18 months	5	2
18 months–2 years	3	0
2–2½ years	2	1
2½–3 years	1	1
3–4 years	2	0

(3) Length of separation

Similarly length of separation can be plotted as shown on Table 13.

Length of separation correlated with the patient group at a 5 per cent level, namely + 0.2380.

Table 13

Length of Separation Related to Patient/Control Groups

Length of Separation	*Patient*	*Control*
Prolonged	3	1
Under 6 months	1	0
Under 1 month	2	2
Under 2 weeks	7	1
Under 1 week	5	4
Total	18	8

(4) Type of separation experience

Consideration was given to the type of separation, that is to say whether overtly traumatic to the child or not, and this was broken down on the Holerith sorter, the results being shown in Table 14.

Table 14

Type of Separation Experience related to Patient/Control Group

Type of Experience	*Patient*	*Control*
1. No separation	32	42
2. Short separation No problems	8	3
3. Long separation No problems	4	2
4. Traumatic separation but no problems	1	0
5. Traumatic separation creating problems	3	2
6. Satisfactory separation but traumatic effect	2	1
Total	50	50

(5) Attempted suicide

Finally in this series consideration was given to those patients who had made suicide attempts and this was related to early separation experiences. Ten patients had attempted suicide. Eight of these had had no separation experience, and of the two who had been separated there had been no problem.

(6) Diagnostic categories

The patients were then broken down into diagnostic categories in order to ascertain if this factor was related to the various aspects of the separation experience. This is shown in Tables 15 and 16.

From the correlation matrix positive correlations are found relating diagnostic categories to separation experiences as follows:

(*a*) Separation experiences with

personality disorder	+ 0.2208 (5 per cent significance)
ideas of reference	+ 0.2810 (1 per cent significance)
delusions	+ 0.3188 (0.1 per cent significance)

(*b*) Length of separation with

patient/control	+ 0.2380 (5 per cent)
schizophrenia	+ 0.2842 (1 per cent)
ideas of reference	+ 0.2511 (1 per cent)
delusions	+ 0.2842 (1 per cent)

(*c*) Bad cover with

schizophrenia + 0.4225 (0.1 per cent)

(*d*) Traumatic effect of separation with

schizophrenia + 0.2703 (1 per cent)

Table 15

Age of Separation Related to Initial Diagnosis

Diagnosis	*Age of Separation (years)*							
	None	*<0.5*	*<1*	*<1.5*	*<2*	*<2.5*	*<3*	*<4*
None	42	0	4	2	0	1	1	0
Schizophrenia	4	1	0	3	2	0	1	0
Depression	5	0	1	0	0	0	0	1
Hysterical	6	0	0	0	0	0	0	0
Anxiety state	6	1	0	1	1	1	0	0
Reactive depression	6	1	0	0	0	0	0	0
Personality disorder	6	1	0	0	0	1	0	0
Obsessional	0	0	0	1	1	0	0	0

Table 16

Tyde of Separation Related to Initial Diagnosis

Diagnosis	*Type of separation (as in Table 14)*					
	None (1.)	*2.*	*3.*	*4.*	*5.*	*6.*
None	42	3	2	0	2	1
Schizophrenia	4	2	1	1	1	2
Depression	5	2	0	0	0	0
Hysterical	6	0	0	0	0	0
Anxiety state	6	3	1	0	0	0
Reactive depression	6	1	0	0	0	0
Personality disorder	6	0	1	0	1	0
Obsessional	0	0	1	0	1	0

(*e*) When age of separation experience is examined in relation to diagnosis some interesting trends emerge. Thus if separation experiences of under the age of 18 months are considered, positive correlations are found with anxiety states at a level of + 0.1574 for 6 months to 1 year, and + 0.2199 (5 per cent level of significance) for under 6 months with childhood neurotic traits. At about 18 months symptoms of thought disorder begin to show positive correlations; thus, delusions + 0.1642, and at age 18 months to 3 years delusions show a positive correlation of 0.3244 (0.1 per cent) with separation experiences. Ideas of reference correlate at + 0.1901. Personality disorder correlates at + 0.2254 (5 per cent).

In the age range 3–6 years the correlation with schizophrenia is + 0.3160 (0.1 per cent), and with depression is + 0.2633 (1 per cent).

With separations occurring over this age the correlation with schizophrenia is +0.3408 (0.1 per cent), and with obsessional states is + 0.2303 (5 per cent).

When an adjustment was made for I.Q. to relate mental age rather than chronological age of separation to diagnosis, the results were as follows:

At M.A. < 18 months the correlation with childhood neurotic traits is + 0.2766 (5 per cent), and with delusions is + 0.3425 (3 per cent).

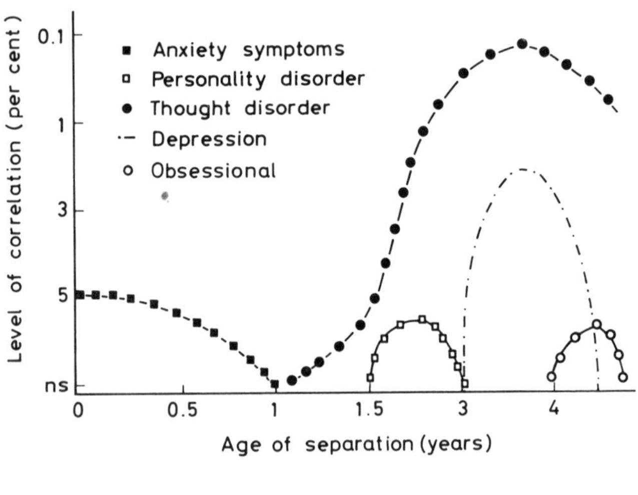

Figure 1 Relationship of diagnosis to age of separation experience

At M.A. 18 months to 3 years the correlation does not reach a significant level.

At M.A. > 3 years the correlation with delusions is 0.2735 (5 per cent).

This can be shown graphically as in *Figure 1*.

(7) Personality traits

Finally separation experiences were related to personality traits and the following positive correlations were found.

(*a*) Separation experience to

childhood neuroticism	+ 0.2064 (5 per cent)
patient's rating scale	+ 0.2826 (1 per cent)
family history	+ 0.2044 (5 per cent)

(*b*) Length of separation to

patient's rating scale	+ 0.3402 (0.1 per cent)

(*c*) Traumatic separation experience to

aggressive traits	+ 0.2937 (1 per cent)

(*d*) Taking separation by age of experience the following correlations were found:

< 6 months to neurosis in childhood
+ 0.2199 (5 per cent)

18 months–3 years to family history
+ 0.1776 (n.s.)
to patient's rating scale
+ 0.2038 (5 per cent)
to I.Q.
+ 0.2444 (< 5 per cent)

3–6 years to family history
+ 0.2280 (5 per cent)
to patient's rating scale
+ 0.3028 (1 per cent).

DISCUSSION

Many studies have considered critical periods of separation from the mother figure in childhood. A few have been quoted in the historical survey (Spitz and Wolf, 1946; Bowlby, 1951; Yarrow, 1961, etc.). In this study separation has therefore been considered by age, length of separation experience, and degree of trauma.

Firstly it has been shown that the patient group has a significantly higher incidence of separation experience of all types, than does the control. From Table 12 it will be seen that the age of separation is fairly evenly divided, but that a positive correlation with adolescent breakdown is found in those aged between 18 months and 3 years.

Most of the separations were between a week and a month in duration. Only four were of the prolonged deprivation type discussed by Bowlby (1951). Again the longer separations were found significantly more commonly in the patient group.

Surprisingly there was no relationship between the separated group and the occurrence of a suicide attempt.

A significant positive correlation was found between a separation experience and the development of personality disorder, and also schizophrenia. In schizophrenia this was particularly so for the longer and more traumatic types of separation experience. It should be noted however that this included two adopted children where in effect there had been a change of mother image entirely at possibly a critical age. However these findings do support those of Goldfarb (1943).

Interesting possibilities concerning analytical theories open up when diagnostic categories are studied, though the numbers are not really large enough to draw valid conclusions. There is a tendency nevertheless as shown in *Figure 1*, for early separations to relate to anxiety symptoms; for separations in the 18 months–4 years group to produce psychoses and to a lesser extent personality disorders, these latter particularly in the 18 months–3 years group, with depression in the 3–4 year group, and finally for obsessional traits to be associated with separation in the > 4-year-olds to a level of 5 per cent significance. The numbers however make these last figures of dubious validity.

When personality traits are considered, a separation experience is seen to relate to childhood neuroticism and to a positive family history at the 5 per cent level, and a traumatic separation experience showed a 1 per cent significance with aggressive traits in personality. Neuroses in childhood were particularly common in those separated under 6 months of age. A relationship with a lowered I.Q. was found in the 18 months–3-year-old group when they had had a separation experience.

The rating scale designed to show up personality defects in the patient's adjustment (as judged by the patient) showed a positive correlation (i.e. poor personality adjustment) with separation experiences in general, to length of separation, and in particular to separation in the > 18 months group.

There was no positive correlation between separation experiences and any of the other items studied.

In terms of total numbers, 16 per cent of the control group had had a separation experience. This compares with Douglas *et al.* (1958) who found that while 50 per cent of the population had been briefly separated before the age of 6 years, only 14 per cent had had a separation measurable in weeks.

The question of age of separation has been considered in the historical survey. Earle and Earle (1961), and Pringle *et al.* (1960) believed that young separations related to personality disorder. Language and abstract functioning may be affected in separations in the < 2 year group. In this study a lower I.Q. was found in those separated in the 18 months–3-year-old group. Possibly the disturbance in abstract functioning in this group may cause a tendency towards thought disorder and schizophrenic symptoms in the adolescent, but this is conjectural.

Although suicide attempt did not relate to separation, it did relate to personality traits of moodiness and anxiety (see Table 20). Ten cases (i.e. 20 per cent) had made an attempt (cf. Balser and Masterson, 1959). There was no correlation with diagnosis.

III. TRAUMATIC EXPERIENCES IN CHILDHOOD

It will be apparent from the above results that not all separation experiences appear traumatic, at any rate on the surface. Equally there will be traumatic experiences other than separation which may affect personality and subsequent breakdown. An attempt was therefore made to quantify the concept of childhood traumatic experience from details of the early history, including separation experiences, terrifying episodes and disturbed relationships with parents (e.g. alcoholism, incest, etc.). These were then merely itemized on a yes–no basis and related to diagnosis and to personality traits. Two groups of individuals could thus be formed—those with an abnormal early history and those without. Similarly the presence of childhood neurosis and other aspects of the child's early life could be related to personality type and diagnostic grouping. The results of these investigations are shown in this section, considering firstly childhood trauma.

Table 17

Relationship of Traumatic Events to Diagnosis

Diagnosis	*Trauma positive*	*Trauma negative*
None	18	32
Schizophrenia	5	5
Depressive	3	4
Hysterical	5	1
Anxiety state	7	3
Reactive depression	3	4
Personality disorder	6	2
Obsessional	2	0

A X^2 test on the total figures of childhood trauma to patient/control = 5.720 which is significant at the 0.02 level of significance (i.e. a 1:50 chance).

Similarly the presence of childhood neurotic traits can be related to diagnosis.

Table 18

Childhood Neurotic Traits to Diagnosis

Diagnosis	*Neurotic Features Positive*	*Neurotic Features Negative*
None	16	34
Schizophrenia	3	7
Depressive	3	4
Hysterical	3	3
Anxiety state	5	5
Reactive depression	4	3
Personality disorder	5	3
Obsessional	0	2

A X^2 test here on the total numbers neurosis/patient–control = 1.500 is not significant.

On the correlation matrix childhood neurosis correlates

with	separation at	+ 0.2064	(5 per cent)
and with	sibling order	+ 0.1487	(< 5 per cent level)
	family history	+ 0.2739	(1 per cent)
	inadequate mothering	+ 0.2505	(≏ 1 per cent)
	abnormal early history	+ 0.3941	(0.1 per cent)
	poor mother–adolescent relationship	+ 0.2104	(5 per cent)
	personality disorder	+ 0.2188	(5 per cent).

The question of phobic symptoms will now be considered.

It was noted in the two correlation matrices that phobias, unlike other symptoms, showed no difference between the patient and control groups. A phobia here is defined as a morbid fear of some situation or object, distinguishing it from the psychoneurotic illness of phobic anxiety state. Monosymptomatic phobias were as common in the control group as in the patient group, and in fact the presence of a phobia correlated with a good prognosis in Matrix A at a level of 0.2932 which is a 1 per cent level of significance, and in Matrix B showed a correlation of 0.3110 at the 5 per cent level of significance. The only other positive correlation was with the patient's total adequate relationships at follow-up, where phobias had a positive correlation of 0.2935 (at a 5 per cent level), a result of dubious relevence.

A breakdown of the phobias is shown in Table 19 where it will

Table 19

Type of Phobia and Precipitant

Phobia	*Patient*	*Control*	*Known Precipitant Patient*	*Known Precipitant Control*
The dark	15	15	6	5
Heights	11	16	3	2
Being alone	13	11	3	0
Being shut in or confined	1	3	1	0
People—crowds	7	1	0	0
Thunder	1	2	0	0
Insects, etc.	4	2	0	0
Others	14	12	4	6

Table 20

Correlation Results Relating Personality to Early Experience

Personality Trait	*Correlation Item*	*Correlation*	*Level of Significance (per cent)*
Aggressiveness	Schizophrenia	+ 0.2937	1
	Family history mental illness	+ 0.2454	3
	Abnormal early history	+ 0.2335	3
	Poor total adequate relationships	+ 0.2171	5
	Bad father relationship	+ 0.2266	5
	Bad effect of separation experience	+ 0.2703	1
	Separation > 4 years	+ 0.3408	0.1
	Bad prognosis	+ 0.3923	0.1
Obsessionality	Separation > 4 years	+ 0.2303	3
Anxiety	Suicide attempt	+ 0.4001	0.1
	Poor mother–child relationship	+ 0.3647	0.1
	Poor father relationship	+ 0.2406	3
	Abnormal early history	+ 0.1712	n.s.
	Separation experience	—	
	Bad prognosis	+ 0.3122	0.1
Moodiness	Suicide attempt	+ 0.4001	0.1
	Total adequate relationships	− 0.2340	3
	Poor mother relationship	+ 0.3171	0.1
	Poor father relationship	+ 0.2138	5

n.s. not significant

Table 21

Correlation Results Relating Early Relationships and Symptomatology

Correlates		*Correlation*	*Significance (per cent)*
Abnormal early history	to patient/control	+ 0.2170	5
	to personality disorder	+ 0.2242	5
	to aggressiveness	+ 0.2335	5
	to family history	+ 0.2097	5
	to poor total relationships	+ 0.2556	1
	to self-rating	+ 0.2798	1
Good mother–child relationship	to male child, i.e. sex	+ 0.2233	5
	to patient/control	− 0.3677	0.1
	to personality disorder	− 0.3922	0.1
	to mood disturbance	− 0.3029	1
	to anxiety	− 0.3647	0.1
	to moodiness	− 0.3171	0.1
	to childhood neurosis	− 0.2104	5
	to abnormal early history	− 0.2538	1
	to patient self-rating	− 0.4254	0.1
	to father–child relationship	− 0.4493	0.1
	to bad prognosis	− 0.3138	0.1
Good father–child relationship	to patient/control	− 0.3118	0.1
	to personality disorder	− 0.2602	1
	to mood disorder	− 0.2283	5
	to self-rating	− 0.5257	0.1

be seen that three items occur much more commonly. This is no doubt partly because these were the items cited as examples in the questionnaire.

The total number of patients with phobias was 39, and controls 35. Of the 'others' group, items included dogs, water, lifts, fears of death, loud noises, and a few specific unusual items directly related to a known earlier traumatic event.

Fears of the dark often dated back to babyhood. One case followed separation at 3 years for tonsillectomy. Another was accidentally locked alone in the dark as a small child for some hours. In two cases the mother suffered from the same fear. Fears of the dark often followed a separation experience, and in three cases the fear followed being isolated in the dark as a punishment. However, in many cases there was no retrospectively identifiable trigger to the phobia. This, of course, does not prove that such did not exist. Further, there often appeared to be a traumatic event followed by anxiety which crystallized on to a specific situational phobia which might be postulated to have coincidentally been present at the time.

Of those patients who feared heights, a few identified a fall as triggering this off.

If separation experiences are compared with phobias in general, there is no significant correlation, but if fears of the dark are considered, there is a relationship with separation at the 0.1 level of significance.

A X^2 test for fear of heights, and fear of being alone, compared with separation showed no significance.

Finally in this section the correlation matrix results relating personality traits to trauma will be summarized. They are set out in Table 20.

Table 21 shows a comparison of abnormal early history and parent relationships to personality aspects.

DISCUSSION

Bowlby (1946) has established that certain personality defects may be the result of childhood deprivation or trauma—though usually of the grosser kind.

With regard to critical ages, Spitz and Wolf (1946) have shown that the crucial age for a child to start developing true object relations was in the 3–6 months age group.

It can be surmized from the work of Hebb (1949), Corner (1944) and Erikson (1959), that it is probable that the arresting of this development at a critical age can permanently prevent the child's proper subsequent emotional development. Early trauma may produce widespread general disturbance. Later trauma may produce more localized problems. It is possible that *Figure 1* is representing this in simple form.

It seems that a more complete deprivation produces an asocial character: an ambivalent antisocial character is produced by the interspersal of satisfaction and deprivation.

The first part of this section considers the relationship of childhood trauma, quantified in the manner described, to other items. A separation experience is in this context one aspect of a traumatic childhood.

Table 17 establishes that there is a significant increase in childhood trauma in the patient group ($P = 0.02$). Childhood neuroticism is not different between patient and control groups however. There is nevertheless a relationship between neuroticism in childhood and an abnormal early history on the correlation matrix ($+ 0.3941 = 0.1$ per cent significant level) and a smaller but still significant correlation with inadequate mothering, a positive family history, and subsequent personality disorder.

When separate personality traits are considered significant differences are found in the traits concerned with mixing with others, but these are not related to the kind of separation experiences that are being considered.

A positive correlation was identified however between fears of the dark and a separation experience. One might postulate that the separation was more keenly felt in the darkness, and that at night-time fears of further separation were reinforced by being left alone on return from this separation experience.

Tables 20 and 21 which relate personality traits to aspects of trauma and to diagnosis show that aggressiveness correlates with an abnormal early history and with a bad father relationship, with separation in the older group and in particular those separations where there had been a particularly traumatic effect on the child at the time. Obsessionality also related to separation.

Anxiety, however, was related to poor mother–child relationships ($P = 0.001$) but also to poor father relationships and abnormal early history. It was not related to a separation experience. Moodiness also related to poor early parental relationships.

These findings suggest that personality traits may be influenced by early environment. Difficulty with mother gives anxiety, difficulty with father aggression, or perhaps the differing ages at which mother and father take on importance is the more critical factor when relating this to a separation experience.

Looked at the other way round, as in Table 21, an abnormal early history distinguishes patients from controls ($r = 0.2170$). It is found in personality disorders, aggressive personalities, and shows itself later in an inability to make good personal relationships and a tendency to think poorly of oneself, i.e. a lack of self-confidence This ties in with many of Bowlby's ideas.

Disturbed mother–child relationships were found in personality disorders, in anxiety and moodiness, in a proneness to childhood neurotic traits and to a lack of self-confidence in adolescence. Disturbed father–child relationships had an even stronger relationship to loss of self-confidence and a poor self-rating ($r = -0.5257$, $P = 0.1$ per cent). Mood disorder and personality disorder were also related. Mathis (1964) found an association with a poor father relationship and delinquent behaviour.

We find therefore a number of relatively non-specific factors to be associated with subsequent personality breakdown. These include elements of separation experiences, abnormal early history, trauma and disturbance in parental relationships. Quantified, these show statistically significant relationships with the patient group. Lewis (1954) also found a variety of factors to be important. She found that parental rejection led to aggressive behaviour, and a repressive regime to neurosis. To disentangle all these factors—separation, age of trauma, severity in length and degree, parental relationships and all the other ramifications, is probably an impossible task. It is only by quantifying that the total significance of these events on the subsequent personality and adjustment can be appreciated, since to take one item in isolation is to ignore many other possible significant variables. However, as Yarrow (1961) pointed out, the attempt must be made, and in a small way in this section, this has been attempted.

IV. THE CONCEPT OF TOTAL ADEQUATE RELATIONSHIPS

It has been the author's contention that many patients have, for one reason or another, a dearth of satisfactory human relationships, on which they can depend. It was hypothesized that the patient group would show significantly fewer of these relationships than a control group and that those with the poorest relationships would have the poorest prognosis, other things being equal. It was hoped

Table 22

T.A.R. Scale, Comparison of Patient and Control Groups

		Patient	*Control*
T.A.R. Score*	9	12	29
	7	5	2
	5	12	10
	3	7	3
	1	14	6
Total		50	50

* N.B. on this table, 9 is the best score

Table 23

Relationship of Final Diagnostic Formulation to Initial T.A.R. Score

T.A.R. (1)	9 7 1	1 3 1	1 5 3	1 7 9	5 5 1	5 5 9
Final diagnosis*	2 9 8	2 8 4	4 9 8	8 4 2	8 7 8	5 7 5
T.A.R. (1)	9 1 3	9 5 7	1 9 1	3 7 7	3 5 5	1 5 9
Final diagnosis	8 2 8	8 5 8	8 7 7	5 3 3	8 8 8	7 2 7
T.A.R. (1)	1 1 9	9 5 5	1 9 5	3 3 9	9 1	
Final diagnosis	8 8 5	5 8 8	2 4 7	7 2 5	8 2	

* Diagnostic key; 2 = schizophrenia; 3 = endogenous depression; 4 = hysterical reaction; 5 = anxiety state; 7 = depressive reaction; 8 = personality disorder; 9 = obsessional state

Table 24

Significant Correlations Found Relating to T.A.R. Score

Item	*Correlation*	*Significance (per cent)*
Patient/control	+ 0.3329	0.1
Personality disorder	+ 0.2751	1.0
Schizophrenia	+ 0.1935	5.0
Depressive reaction	+ 0.2187	5.0
Abnormal early history	+ 0.2556	1
Moodiness	+ 0.2340	5
Aggressiveness	+ 0.2171	5

to show that where a satisfactory psychotherapeutic relationship had been made in these cases, that the prognosis could be improved.

That this concept is plausible has been shown by Bowlby's work and his concept of the affectionless character (Bowlby, 1951).

The type of relationship which the author had in mind was one in which an empathetic relationship existed, of mutual trust, confidence and support, allowing security to develop as the individual grew up. This relationship might exist with parents, siblings, close friends or relatives, or figures outside the immediate circle such as church or youth leaders, doctors and so on.

In an attempt to quantify these relationships, each individual in the survey was asked about the number of relationships of this type that they had, who they were, and how secure they felt the relationship to be. This was then scored on a rating scale to form a quantitative measure. This scale was compared with other items in the individual's personality, the possible psychopathological features in the history, and in the patient group, with prognosis. For convenience this scale will be referred to as 'T.A.R.' (total adequate relationships).

A further assessment of this T.A.R. scale was made on the patient group at two year follow-up review, and a second T.A.R. (2) score produced for comparison with the first.

Consideration is first given to a comparison of the T.A.R. scale between control and patient groups. This is set out in Table 22.

If this is split between those with good relationships (score 5 or more) and those poorer (score 3 or less), and a X^2 test performed, $X^2 = 5.74$ where $P \simeq 0.02$ which is a highly significant finding.

A consideration is given to a comparison of diagnosis with the T.A.R. score in Table 23.

Here it will be seen that the personality disorders score 77 out of a possible score of 171, and the schizophrenics 30 out of a possible 72. The anxiety states however score 49 out of a possible 63. The T.A.R. score bore no relationship to suicide attempt.

A consideration of the correlations obtained on the first matrix shows the results given in Table 24.

DISCUSSION

The concept of 'total adequate relationships' was devised out of the work of Bowlby (1951) and his concept of the affectionless character. Diagnosis in this age group has been shown often to be meaningless and it is probable that in adolescence many of the breakdowns seen are patterns resultant upon previous experience, combined with the trigger of an adolescent crisis, (Masterson *et al.*, 1966) in some shape or form. That the ability to relate, and to confide, might be important in causation and in prognosis has been emphasized. In this section an attempt has been made to quantify and measure this concept to show a correlation between it and the other items in the matrix.

It will be seen from Table 22 that the T.A.R. score in the patient group is generally lower than that of the controls, and indeed a X^2 test shows this to be significant at a level of $P = 0.02$. The scale thus distinguishes the two groups.

When diagnosis is considered the average T.A.R. score for a control is 6.8. The score for personality disorder is 4.0, schizophrenia 3.75, but for anxiety state is 7.0 which is as good as, and in fact slightly better than, that of controls. Depression also scores 7.0, but depressive reactions 4.75; hysteria scores 4.5 and obsessionals 6.

The numbers for depression and obsessionals are small, but generally the anxiety states, endogenous depressions and obsessionals did not differ from controls in terms of total adequate relationships. Personality disorders, reactive depressions and schizophrenia were grouped together however in being at least 3 points lower than the others.

The scatter, however, in these scores makes the s.d. and s.e. such that with these numbers the results cannot be said quite to reach statistical significance in this regard, if individual diagnoses are taken separately.

The results of the correlation matrix confirm at a significance of 0.1 per cent ($r = +0.3329$) the difference between patient and control groups. This difference appears to be marked in personality disorders and schizophrenia, in the former at a 1 per cent level, in the latter and in depressive reactions at a 5 per cent level.

The T.A.R. score did not show a significant correlation with separation experience nor a poor mother–child relationship. It correlated with the personality traits of moodiness and aggression, but interestingly did correlate with abnormal early history at a 1 per cent level. Since 'abnormal early history' was a scale derived from separation experiences and poor mother relationships, and in addition, childhood neuroses and problems to do with relating to others in childhood, it suggests that these latter features are important in producing a positive correlation, and that these problems are continued into adolescence to form the basis of a difficulty in relating, and the eventual presence of a personality disorder in the adolescent.

The T.A.R. score did not correlate significantly with suicide attempt, nor with the other scales itemized in the matrix.

V. RELATIONSHIP THERAPY

Differing schools of thought have had differing ideas with regard to the theoretical implications of psychotherapy, from orthodox Freudian analytical concepts at one extreme to behaviourist concepts at the other. It is however on the basis of a relationship of empathetic type that psychotherapy obtains its results, and whether one considers this as due to a classic transference relationship or to a learning theory effect with relief of anxiety and increasing security in an empathetic milieu is perhaps not too important in practical terms.

On the question of personality problems and other adolescent disorders it has equally been shown that lack of these relationships in children can lead to later problems and the type of 'affectionless character' described by Bowlby (1951). These problems have been brought out in the historical survey (Levy, 1937; Powdermaker *et al.*, 1937; Goldfarb, 1943), and have also been apparent in that section of the results in this book dealing with the concept of 'total adequate relationships'.

On this basis, therefore, an attempt has been made to establish whether therapy, during which an empathetic relationship had been established with the patient, could be shown to give benefit to those cases in particular where a T.A.R. score was initially low, and whether in these cases the second T.A.R. score would show, in the patient's view, a measurable improvement. There is evidence to suggest that in a previous series of adolescents where this technique has been adopted the results have been promising (Aubry, 1955). In this type of therapy with adolescents one is not so much a father as a big brother or even a kind of boyfriend image, a hero figure—but the all-important thing is the quality of the confidence and empathy achieved. This therapy has been described as 'relationship therapy'. In this series of 50 cases certain patients, due to circumstances in the timing, diagnosis or environmental situation generally, lent themselves to this kind of therapy. These cases were personally followed up in therapy over a minimum 2 year (maximum 5 year) period and came to relate to the therapist in a strongly empathetic way, apparently acquiring much support from the relationship. This type of therapy applied to 20 of the 50 cases. The results of this part of the study are now presented.

Table 25

Comparisons of T.A.R. Scales, F.A.R. Scale, Separations, Trauma and Relationship Therapy

Patient number	*1*	*2*	*3*	*4*	*5*	*6*	*7*	*8*	*9*	*10*	*11*	*12*	*13*	*14*	*15*	*16*	*17*	*18*	*19*	*20*	*21*	*22*	*23*	*24*	*25*
Traumatic separation	+	−	−	+	+	−	−	+	−	−	−	−	−	−	−	−	+	−	−	−	−	−	−	−	+
T.A.R. (1)	9	7	1	1	3	1	1	5	3	1	7	9	5	5	1	5	5	9	9	1	3	9	5	7	1
T.A.R. (2)	4	8	8	4	4	4	8	6	4	4	4	6	2	6	2	8	6	4	8	4	6	4	8	6	6
Relationship therapy given	+	+	* +	+	* +	+	+	+	* +	* +	−	+	* −	−	* −	* −	−	* +	* −	−	* −	* −	−	−	* −
Final adjustment rating (F.A.R.)	3	1	1	3	2	3	1	2	2	2	2	3	4	2	1	2	2	2	2	4	2	3	2	1	1

Patient number	*26*	*27*	*28*	*29*	*30*	*31*	*32*	*33*	*34*	*35*	*36*	*37*	*38*	*39*	*40*	*41*	*42*	*43*	*44*	*45*	*46*	*47*	*48*	*49*	*50*
Traumatic separation	−	−	−	−	−	+	−	−	−	−	−	−	−	−	−	−	−	−	−	−	−	−	−	−	+
T.A.R. (1)	9	1	3	7	7	3	5	5	1	5	9	1	1	9	9	5	5	1	9	5	3	3	9	9	1
T.A.R. (2)	8	6	4	8	6	8	2	4	8	8	4	4	4	6	8	4	4	6	6	4	2	8	8	4	6
Relationship therapy given	+	−	+	−	−	* +	* −	* −	−	−	+	* −	* −	−	+	* +	* +	−	−	+	−	−	−	* −	−
Final adjustment rating (F.A.R.)	1	2	4	1	2	1	3	3	1	1	3	2	2	1	2	2	2	4	3	3	2	1	1	1	3

* = Diagnosis of personality disorder

Table 25 compares those patients who received relationship therapy, those who had a traumatic separation experience, and the first and second T.A.R. ratings. It also records the final adjustment rating at two year follow-up on the 50 patients. This latter rating was an attempt to quantify improvement and is described in the section on material and method.

In this table a score of 9 in the T.A.R. scale is a maximally good score. A score of 1 is a minimally poor score. The final adjustment rating is scored 1 to 4; the higher the score the poorer is the patient's performance on this scale.

A consideration of this table shows that the patients with a traumatic separation experience fared somewhat worse in terms of T.A.R. ratings than did the rest. An improvement in relationships was claimed by the patients in 29 cases. Twenty-one said their personal relationships were if anything worse. Of those who had had

Table 26

Positive Correlations referring to T.A.R. Scores and a Response to Relationship Therapy

Item	*Correlate*	*Correlation*	*Significance (per cent)*
T.A.R. (1)	Re-admissions	− 0.3367	3
	Anxiety	− 0.2649	≏5
	T.A.R. (2)	− 0.1053	n.s.
	No other correlations were significant		
T.A.R. (2)	Residual symptoms	− 0.3999	1
	Final prognosis	+ 0.4115	1
	Patients' final view of themselves	+ 0.3528	1
	Relationship therapy	− 0.0708	n.s.
	No other correlations were significant		
Relationship therapy	I.Q.	− 0.4194	1
	Follow-up	+ 0.3275	3
	Separation age 18 months–3 years	+ 0.3118	5
	No other correlations were significant		

n.s. not significant

the presumed benefit of relationship therapy (total 20) 11 said they had better personal relationships, and 9 were if anything worse. In 9 cases therefore a good relationship with the therapist had not had a good effect on relationships overall, and 18 had improved in this respect without this kind of therapy. These differences are not significant. The final adjustment rating demonstrated that 15 had a poor adjustment, 15 a good adjustment, and 20 a reasonable adjustment in terms of that which the scale set out to measure. Of the 20 who had received 'relationship therapy', 5 had a good adjustment, 8 reasonable, and 7 poor. Those who had and those who had not had relationship therapy therefore show no difference in terms of the final adjustment rating, if taken as a group.

Table 26 shows the results of the computer analysis.

Thus there was no correlation between T.A.R. scores and separation, or other aspects of early history, nor did relationship therapy demonstrably improve prognosis in the total group.

DISCUSSION

It was hoped in this investigation to show that a certain type of psychotherapy aimed at creating a confiding relationship with the patient which would compensate for a low T.A.R. score, would improve prognosis in so far as it was successful. From this relationship the adolescent might learn to improve his relationship with others.

Powdermaker *et al.* (1937) showed 50 per cent good results in this type of patient, the response relating to abnormal early history, but not to I.Q. or inheritance. Bowlby (1951) felt the affectionless character to be a difficult problem since the psychiatrist was robbed of his best tool, namely the ability to relate. Aubry (1955) produced good results nevertheless in this group.

Table 25 considers aspects of this concept. The mean T.A.R. (1) score of those traumatically separated was 3.1. In those who subsequently received relationship therapy the mean was 4.8 which is the mean for the patient group as a whole. Of the personality disorders the 8 who received relationship therapy had a mean T.A.R. (1) of 3.75, and those not so treated a mean of 4.5. The final T.A.R. (2) score in the treated group was 5.0 (an improvement of 1.25) and in the non-treated 4.5 (no improvement). Unfortunately, these figures do not achieve statistical significance if a t-test is performed to compare the significance of the difference between the means, but the trend is apparent and implies that relationship therapy in this group is a desirable method of therapy. Improvement in other diagnostic categories showed no difference between the relationship therapy group and the rest.

When the results of the matrix are considered, these with a good T.A.R. (1) score are seen to fare better in terms of re-admissions than did those with a poor score. Similarly, the T.A.R. (2) score correlated with lack of residual symptoms at a 1 per cent level. Those with a good T.A.R. (2) score had a better prognosis and felt themselves to be improved though the scale did not correlate significantly with relationship therapy when applied to the group as a whole.

VI. PROGNOSTIC INDICATORS

It will be recalled that it was hoped to be able to identify prognostic indicators in the data collected. To this end, an assessment was made at the two year follow-up of the outcome of the original illness and the present situation of the patient. Various aspects of their functioning were rated as described in the section on material and method, and a rating scale devised to assess final adjustment. These items could then be compared with the original rating scales concerned with items in the early history, adequacy of mothering, and the patient's previous personality and stability, including the T.A.R. score. These items could then be compared on the second correlation matrix to see if any of them proved to be of significant prognostic relevance.

Certain statistical procedures are inappropriate to the investigation of these scales since the curves do not follow a curve of normal distribution and the means are 'skewed', due to the scoring of items. X^2 tests and in some instances t-tests can be applied however if the appropriate Fisher's tables are used.

Initially the patient and control groups were compared to consider whether prognostic differences could be found between the two groups. Some of these findings have been discussed under previous headings but are collected together for convenience in Table 27.

The patient and control groups were then compared with regard to the rating scales devised, in an attempt to quantify possible psychopathological aspects of the patient's previous history and adjustment, in the belief that it is the sum total of these adverse factors that will show significance rather than any individual item considered in isolation.

Table 27

Significant Correlations Contrasting Patient/Control Groups

Item	*Correlation*	*Significance (per cent)*
Patient group:		
Family history	+ 0.4104	0.1
Childhood neurosis	n.s.	
Unsatisfactory mother	n.s.	
T.A.R. (1)	− 0.3329	0.1
Abnormal early history	+ 0.2170	5
Self-rating	− 0.4646	0.1
Mother–child poor relationship	+ 0.3677	0.1
Bad father–child relationship	+ 0.3118	0.2
Separation experience	+ 0.2478	≃1
Length of separation	+ 0.2380	3
Age of separation (chronological) 18 months–3 years	+ 0.2676	1

n.s. not significant

Table 28a

Comparison of Rating Scales, Patient Group

Scale	*1*	*2*	*3*	*4*	*A.E.H.*	*T.A.R.* (*1*)	*M.U.R.*
Score							
0	—	—	—	—	—	—	6
1	17	1	34	7	33	14	—
2	1	6	—	13	—	—	25
3	17	13	9	14	16	7	—
4	0	6	—	8	—	—	12
5	4	10	5	5	1	12	—
6	5	8	—	3	—	—	5
7	3	5	2	—	0	5	—
8	2	1	—	—	—	—	2
9	1	0	—	—	—	12	—
10	—	—	—	—	—	—	0
Total	50	50	50	50	50	50	50

Table 28b

Comparison of Rating Scales, Control Group

Scale	*1*	*2*	*3*	*4*	*A.E.H.*	*T.A.R. (1)*	*M.U.R.*
Score							
0	—	—	—	—	—	—	21
1	20	5	46	15	42	6	—
2	0	15	—	27	—	—	23
3	21	15	4	8	8	3	—
4	0	8	—	0	—	—	5
5	3	7	0	0	0	10	—
6	5	0	—	0	—	—	1
7	0	0	0	—	0	2	—
8	1	0	—	—	—	—	0
9	0	0	—	—	—	29	—
10	—	—	—	—	—	—	0
Total	50	50	50	50	50	50	50

Key to Tables 28a and b

Scale 1. This scale was a rating of competence in mothering, as derived from items in the original questionnaires. These scales were merely a measure of the sum of various factors considered of possible relevance, and therefore have no more weight than the relevance of individual items to what was being considered. However, if any significant difference is observed it will be a measure of quantitative differences between the patients' upbringing as a group, and that of the controls.

A low score in this scale (as in all the scales shown here except T.A.R.) indicates a good value—in this case a high standard of mothering which was in the author's opinion shown by the questionnaire—and a high score similarly indicates a bad mother.

Scale 2. This scale attempted to quantify good aspects of the patient's personality and functioning as rated by the author.

Scale 3. This scale similarly considered the adjustment of the child from the parents' viewpoint.

Scale 4. Finally a scale was devised concerning the patient's own opinion of his adjustment and personality.

A.E.H. The A.E.H. score (abnormal early history) was a combination of the following items, each scored if positive, a high score thus indicating a maximally unsatisfactory early life experience.

(*a*) Separation experiences.
(*b*) Poor or absent father.
(*c*) Slow development of milestones.
(*d*) Presence of childhood neuroses.
(*e*) Childhood 'affectionless character'.
(*f*) Poor mothering.
(*g*) Childhood traumas of other types.

The choosing of these items is entirely arbitrary—the important point being whether a difference is shown between the two groups and whether the score has prognostic relevance.

T.A.R. (*1*) *Score.* The 'total adequate relationships' measure. This has been previously described.

M.U.R. Scale. This scale was a 'mutual understanding rating' based on inconsistencies between the answers given to questions by the adolescent and the identical questions asked of the mother. A high score indicates a poor level of confidence between the two.

The following 'Gambolgram' attempts to show these scores in diagramatic form (*Figures 2–8*).

A consideration of these diagrams will show that in every case the control group predominates at the left hand side of the graph and the patient group dominates the higher scoring right hand end of the scale, although in both control and patient groups the highest numbers are always at the low end of the scale, except in the T.A.R. (1).

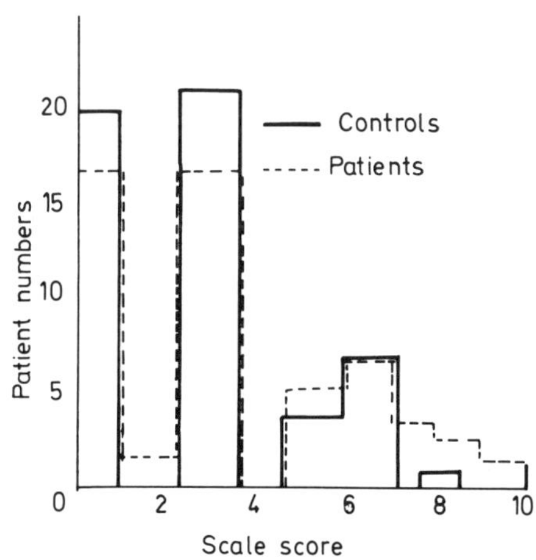

Figure 2 Scale 1—mother competence

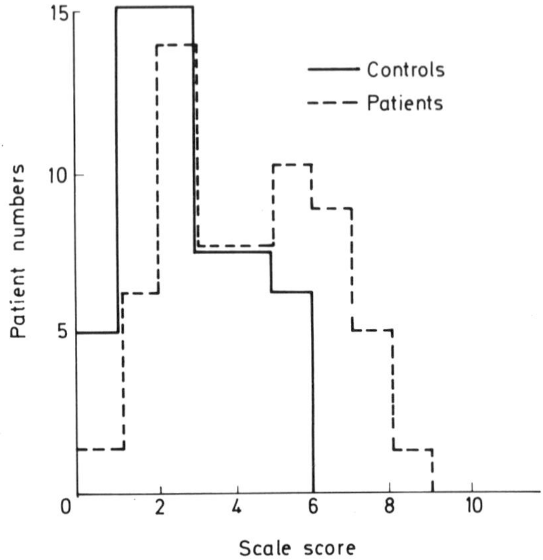

Figure 3 Scale 2—doctor's rating of patient's personality

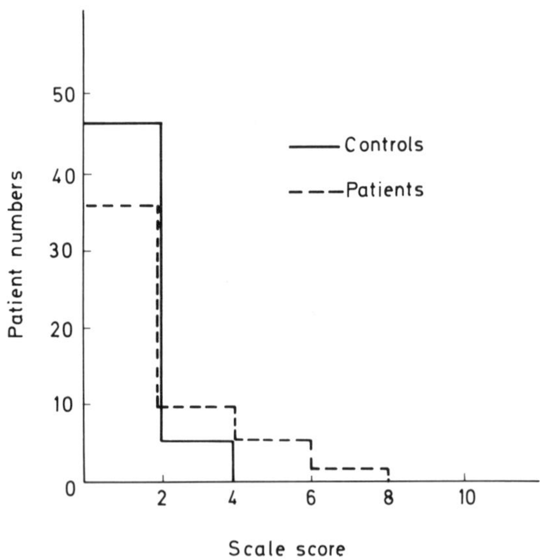

Figure 4 Scale 3—Parents' view of child's adjustment

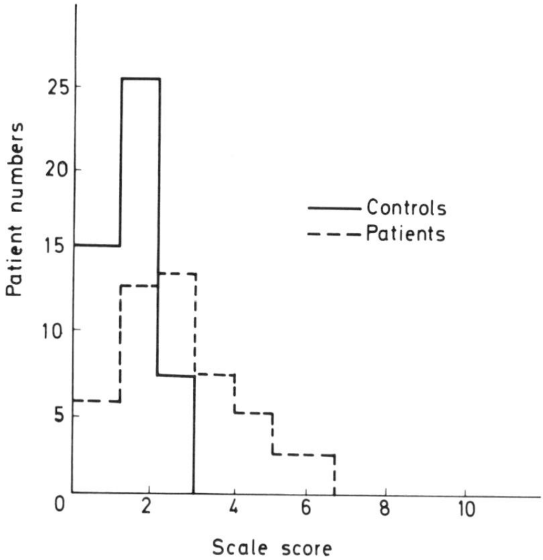

Figure 5 Scale 4—patient's view of personality adjustment

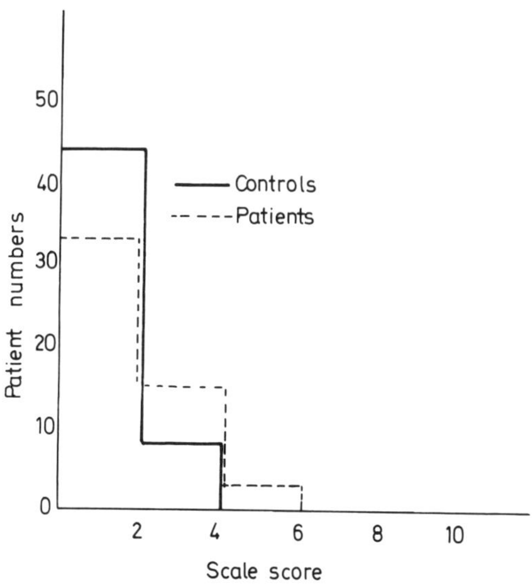

Figure 6 A.E.H.—'abnormal early history' score

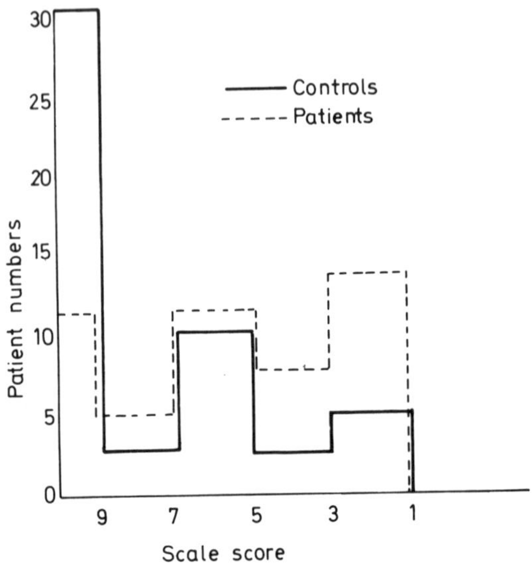

Figure 7 *T.A.R.(1)—the 'total adequate relationships (initial)' measure*

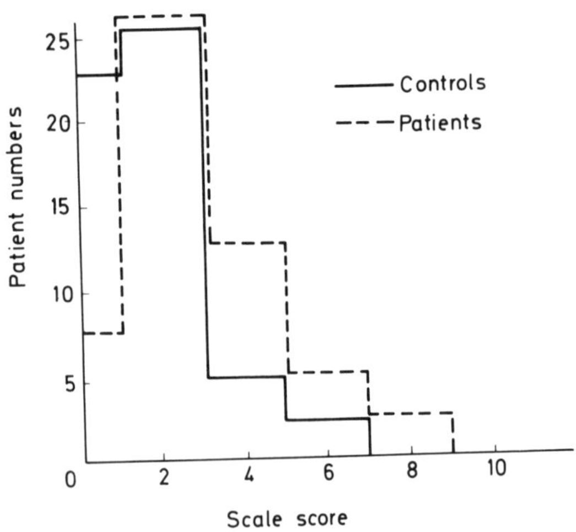

Figure 8 *M.U.R.—the 'mutual understanding rating' scale*

If these tests are subjected to a X^2 test (as described on page 54) by comparing patient with control scores and dividing the scores into 'good' and 'bad' at a given cut-off point as suitable to the scale, the following results emerge:

Figure	Cut-Off Point Score	X^2	P
1	≤ 3	1.38	0.3
2	≤ 5	14.2	< 0.001
3	≤ 3	18.4	< 0.001
4	≤ 2	18.8	< 0.001
A.E.H.	≤ 1	3.42	0.1
T.A.R. (1)	≤ 4	5.75	0.02
M.U.R.	≤ 2	7.65	0.01

Equally, these results can be subjected to a t-test to measure the critical ratio and their significance using the formula

$$t = \frac{\text{mean } 1 - \text{mean } 2}{\text{s.e.}(m - n)}$$

and obtaining P from Fisher's table of t (d.f. = 98) where the significance of the difference between the means of two small uncorrelated samples is tested. (It should be noted here that strictly the samples do not adhere to a normal curve of distribution in the population tested, though the scores are distributed normally around their own means. However, this does not distort the results to a significant degree in this test so that they would be invalid).

The results are as follows:

Figure	t	P
1	1.5	0.10
2	4.3	< 0.001
3	3.4	0.001
4	5.2	< 0.001
A.E.H.	2.2	0.05
T.A.R. (1)	3.7	0.001
M.U.R.	4.2	< 0.001

Thus whichever technique is used these quantitative measures act as distinguishers between patient and control groups at in some cases highly significant levels. Thus the answers of the parents of patients distinguished that their offspring had functioned less satisfactorily in childhood, and that abnormalities in the early history were as a group commoner. Furthermore, the ability of the patients to empathise is shown as clearly deficient when compared with a normal group. Finally, there is a marked difference in the degree of mutual understanding between parent and adolescent in the two groups.

Turning now to the correlation matrix A we may note those items which relate to the prognostic estimate on the patient's discharge after the initial assessment. These are shown in Table 29.

Table 29

Correlations between Prognostic Expectation and Items on Matrix A

Item	*Correlation*	*Significance (per cent)*
Separation experience	—	n.s.
Diagnosis schizophrenia	− 0.4955	0.1
Depressive reaction	− 0.2684	1
Suicide attempt	− 0.2334	5
Aggressive behaviour	− 0.3923	0.1
Anxiety	− 0.3122	0.1
Phobic features	+ 0.2932	1
Family history	− 0.3895	0.1
Patient's rating scale	− 0.5148	0.1
Mother–child relationship	− 0.3138	0.1
Separation experience at > 4 years	− 0.2392	5

Finally, the results of the correlation matrix B are considered. Matrix B referred to the patient group only, and considered the patient's symptomatology and early history of trauma and separation in relation to the two year follow-up findings of 'final outcome', with regard to treatment, progress and final adjustment. In this matrix, since I.Q. was known and adjustment was made so that the age of separation was considered as a mental age rather than a chronological age, in terms of possible 'critical periods,' this was thought on theoretical grounds to be a more relevant figure. This M.A. was obtained by finding the chronological age of separation and then applying the formula M.A. = I.Q. × C.A./100, where M.A. = mental age of separation and C.A. = chronological age of separation.

In this matrix a correlation of > 0.28 = a 5 per cent level of significance; 0.36 = a 1 per cent level, and 0.45 = a 0.1 per cent level.

The results of the two year follow-up are as follows.

It was found that I.Q. correlated with a 'bad' mother at a correlation of − 0.3836, i.e. a 1 per cent level of significance, indicating either that bad mothers cause the child's I.Q. to develop less well—as suggested in work by Goldfarb (1943), or that children with low I.Q.s cause the mothers to become less satisfactory in the the terms under which this conclusion was drawn.

Similarly, I.Q. correlated negatively with the ability to form a relationship with the therapist (r = −0.4194, significance = 1 per cent).

I.Q. also was related at a correlate of 0.2444 (not quite significant at the 5 per cent level) to a separation at the age M.A. = 18 months to 3 years.

Table 30 shows the correlation between symptomatology, i.e. symptom complexes on the lines of Masterson's ideas (Masterson *et al.*, 1963), and subsequent events.

Table 31 shows the correlations between the T.A.R. responses at two year follow-up, transference relationships and residual symptoms.

Table 30

Correlates with Outcome to Symptomatology

Item		*Correlate*	*Significance (per cent)*
Mood disorder	to residual symptoms	+ 0.2548	<5
Obsessions	to re-admission	+ 0.2207	<5
Anxiety	to T.A.R. (1)	+ 0.2649	<5
Phobias	to good prognosis	+ 0.3110	5
,,	to T.A.R. (2)	+ 0.2935	5
Delusions	to family history	+ 0.3825	1
,,	to follow-up	+ 0.3132	5
,,	to re-admissions	+ 0.3013	5
,,	to length of separation	+ 0.2813	5
,,	to age of separation M.A. = < 18 months	+ 0.3425	3
	> 3 years	+ 0.2735	5
Family history	to poor final prognosis	+ 0.2989	5
,,	to good mother	− 0.2826	5

Table 31

Item		*Correlate*	*Significance (per cent)*
T.A.R. (1)	to re-admissions	− 0.3367	3
T.A.R. (2)	to phobias	+ 0.2935	5
,,	to residual symptoms	− 0.3999	1
,,	to final prognosis	+ 0.4115	1
,,	to final patient opinion	+ 0.3528	1
,,	to transference relationship	—	

Finally, Table 32 shows the correlates of significant items relating to final prognosis, re-admissions and final patients' opinions of themselves.

Table 32

Item		*Correlates*	*Significance (per cent)*
Final prognosis	to phobias	+ 0.3110	5
	to family history	− 0.2989	5
	to T.A.R. (2)	+ 0.4115	1
	to separation age M.A. = < 18 months	− 0.2955	5
Re-admissions	to T.A.R. (1)	+ 0.3367	3
	to residual symptoms	+ 0.3544	≏1
	to good prognosis	− 0.3311	3
	to delusions	+ 0.3013	5
	to separation experience	+ 0.3812	1
	at M.A. 18 months –3 years	+ 0.2548	<5
	to final adjustment rating	− 0.3430	3
Final patient opinion	to good mother	+ 0.2837	5
	to T.A.R. (2)	+ 0.3528	≏1
	to separation experience	− 0.2827	5

No other correlates reached a significant level—see Appendix 3B

DISCUSSION

The problem of being able to establish prognostic indicators in adolescent breakdowns is of great importance, especially in view of the unreliability of the diagnoses made, and the critical effect that prognostic indices may have on subsequent careers.

It is known that the prognosis in untreated cases is poor despite some claims to the contrary (Gillespie *et al.*, 1936). The prognosis for psychotics has been established (Carter, 1942) in the pre-drug treatment days, and since. Masterson (1956) comments that little is known about prognosis of adolescent crises. He found that 33 per cent of psychotics did well. Twenty-five per cent of personality disorders did well. One hundred per cent of the anxiety states did well at a > 5 year follow-up.

Phillips (1953) showed that what in effect was a high T.A.R. score correlated with a good prognosis. This was also found to hold true in psychotics (Pitt, 1964). Masterson (1956) found in his study of prognostic indicators that family history and precipitating factors were not relevant in prognosis but a good response to psychotherapy was a good sign in terms of ultimate prognosis.

In this section consideration was first given to those prognostic indicators found in a comparison between the control and patient groups. Table 27 lists these items.

It can be predicted that an adolescent who falls ill is likely to show many of the following features:

1. A positive family history.
2. Poor relationships with friends and relatives in terms of empathy.
3. To have a poor level of confidence in their own ability.
4. To have had problems in early childhood of unspecified type.
5. They are likely to have had disturbed relationships with one or both parents.
6. They will more commonly have been subjected to a separation experience and more particularly a long or traumatic separation experience. This experience is most likely to have occurred in the age group 18 months to 3 years.

These differences are highlighted in the scales which quantify and thus show the total accumulated problems in each individual's childhood. This is shown in *Figures 2–8*. The vertical gives the number of individuals; the horizontal the score on the rating scales. In each case the patients' scores spread along the scale and dominate the higher scoring end of the 'Gambolgram'. The controls all fall at the left hand end of the graph.

The scale concerned with competence of mothering demonstrates that patients have slightly less competent mothers, ($P = 0.13$) as measured by this scale. The second scale, which is the doctor's assessment of previous personality derived from the questionnaire, distinguishes the two groups to a highly significant degree. The parents (scale 3) agreed on this point. So did the adolescents themselves (scale 4). The controls had much better opinions of their earlier personality adjustment than did the patients. The M.U.R. scale was an interesting finding. It was based purely on questions asked of patient and parent about the patient's early history. In some cases the two gave differing answers, e.g. about the presence of a family history, or the presence of an early traumatic experience. This suggested that parent and adolescent did not 'empathize' very highly and the level of confidence between them was low. Those in whom this situation turned out to be present were almost always to be found amongst the patient group. Indeed this item in the history taking proved to be statistically a most significant way of distinguishing the two groups!

Table 29 considers the relationship between the predicted prognosis on discharge and the various personality factors and items of early history included in Matrix A.

The significant correlations are those of diagnostic grouping (schizophrenia, depressive reaction, the presence of a suicide attempt and aggressive behaviour). The presence of anxiety suggested a poor prognosis, but the presence of monosymptomatic phobias was a good sign. A positive family history was a bad sign (cf. Masterson, 1956). The patient's self-rating was a good indicator of immediate post-discharge prognosis. A bad mother–child relationship held a bad prognosis. (All these items had an equal to or better than 1 per cent significance).

Matrix B was then considered. This related to the two year follow-up findings with regard to prognosis and functioning and related this to early history, symptomatology and previous personality. Here no comparison of controls was undertaken.

An interesting finding was that I.Q. related to a poor early mother relationship. This substantiates the views of Goldfarb (1943). This finding reached the 1 per cent level of significance. Again the critical age for separation with regard to a lowering of the I.Q. appeared to be the 18 months to 3 years age group.

Prognosis was related to symptom clusters and diagnostic categories in the expected manner, though only at the 5 per cent level.

However it is probably not realistic to expect a higher correlation with the numbers involved. Phobias again showed a good prognosis. Psychotic illness correlated with re-admissions, and again with separation experiences. The mental age of relevance appeared to be related to separation in the 1 year–18 months M.A. Positive family history related to a bad final prognosis.

It was not possible to draw conclusions concerning the relevance of the mental age concept. This would seem to be a factor worthy of further study but a larger group would be necessary and the I.Q. of controls would need to be known. This was unfortunately impractical in this study.

When T.A.R. scores are considered in relationship to final prognosis, there is a significant negative correlation with re-admissions and a negative correlation at the 1 per cent level with residual symptoms. A good final prognosis related to a high final T.A.R.(2) score at the 1 per cent level ($r = +0.4115$) and to a high level of confidence in the patient with regard to his final opinion of himself. The T.A.R.(2) score did not relate however to the development of a transference type of relationship with the therapist, though this has been elaborated on in the previous section.

A final summary of significant correlations is contained in Table 32. It can be concluded that prognostic indicators can be seen in terms of family history of mental illness, which worsens the prognosis, and similarly a poor ability to empathize as shown in the T.A.R.(2) response. Monosymptomatic phobias do well in terms of final adjustment.

High re-admission rates are related to a poor initial T.A.R.(1) score. They also related to a separation experience at a level of 1 per cent ($r = +0.3812$) particularly at the M.A. of 18 months–3 years.

The patients' final views of themselves in terms of adjustment was related to the original mother–child relationship. A good relationship correlated at the 5 per cent level with a good prognosis. The patients' final opinions also related to a good final T.A.R.(2) score. There was a negative correlation at the 5 per cent level with a separation experience.

No other correlations reached a 5 per cent level of significance. It can be concluded that in terms of good prognosis the ability to relate, the absence of separation, particularly at the 18 months to 3-year-old group, and a good mother–child relationship are important factors. These measures are easy to obtain in a standard interview.

4

CONCLUDING INFERENCES

Earlier in this book we have stated that certain hypotheses were to be tested, namely that (*i*) separation from the mother in early childhood would be commoner in the patient than in the control group. This derived largely from a consideration of the work of Bowlby, Goldfarb and others. It was further thought that it was unlikely that single factors would be responsible for major personality disturbances and that rather a quantitative accumulation or repetition of traumatic factors might be more likely to be found. (*ii*) These traumatic events, measured in a simple quantitative form, might be able to be related to subsequent personality traits and to adolescent breakdown.

These situations might be linked to problems concerned with developing relationships of trust and confidence, initially with parents and later with siblings, and other people with whom the individual might relate, thus perpetuating and worsening the defect. It was postulated therefore (*iii*) that a lack of adequate relationship formation (as measured in a T.A.R. rating) might relate significantly with adolescent illness and prognosis. (*iv*) It was hoped to show that therapy designed deliberately to attempt to fill this need by forming a relationship would improve the prognosis. (*v*) Finally it was hoped to be able to predict prognosis from features in the history and personality of the patient. The conclusions are now set out in summary form.

I. GENERAL INFORMATION

In terms of psychiatric referrals in the Newcastle area, female referrals were nearly twice as common as male.

Initial diagnosis proved as unreliable as many other authors have found it to be, 50 per cent of the original diagnoses having been altered by the end of the follow-up period. This it would seem reflects on the unsatisfactory classification used, whereby conventional adult diagnostic labels are ill suited to adolescent breakdown, rather than a difficulty in delineating symptoms. Much overlap was found in terms of symptom clusters, though it was fairly simple to distinguish disorder of thought, affect and behaviour. Nevertheless even these initial groupings had little predictive value in terms of prognosis.

The final classification was unremarkable and compared with other studies, allowance having been made for the preponderance of females.

Schizophrenia predictably correlated with family history, and this group found it difficult to form good relationships. Anxiety states also showed a positive family history.

Adolescent personality disorders were characterized by a lack of family history, a presence of early childhood neurosis, and a poor T.A.R. score. They had bad relationships with parents, and a high incidence of separation experiences especially at 18 months–3 years. Suicide attempts were common.

A positive family history was significantly commoner in patients than controls. This correlated highly with a bad prognosis.

Only children are more likely to have problems in their early history (i.e. trauma, separation, etc.). To be a middle child appears psychologically safest. Large families were over-represented in the patient group.

II. SEPARATION EXPERIENCES

There is a significantly higher incidence of separation experiences in the patient group than in the control group. This hypothesis has therefore been substantiated. The question of cause and effect is of course a much more difficult one. It seems likely that this is just one 'nail' in the adolescent's eventual 'coffin'. It is possible that the parents of patients were more careful in their recall of these events due to their own guilt feelings, than were the control parents, but this was anticipated and as far as possible eliminated at interview.

Analysing this problem further, it has been shown that the most significant age for separation to occur, in terms of subsequent pathology, is the 18 months–3 years period. The numbers in individual age groupings are however so small as to make these more detailed correlations suspect.

Again in terms of length of separation, the longer the separation, the more likely was the adolescent to appear in the patient rather than the control group, suggesting that the longer the separation, the more pathological it is likely to become.

Further, the more traumatic separations appeared to correlate with certain personality traits and the presence of schizophrenic symptoms.

Suicide attempts did not relate to separation.

Consideration of diagnostic categories shows that separation experiences correlate highly with schizophrenic symptoms, and also with personality disorders. This is also true of the more traumatic and longer separations. Again the numbers are small, and weighted by two adoptions who turned out to be schizophrenic, being counted as a prolonged separation for statistical purposes.

There is suggestive evidence of a splitting into different diagnostic categories or symptom complexes according to the age at which separation occurred. It would appear that early separations tend to correlate with anxiety, leading into personality disturbances in the 18 months age group, followed by thought disorder in those separated in the 18 months–3 years group, psychotic depression also falling in this area, and finally obsessional symptoms in those separated at the 3–6 year age group. Again it must be emphasized that the small numbers make these correlations suspect. Nevertheless the tendency towards this pattern cannot be overlooked.

There was a high correlation between separation and the presence of childhood neuroticism, and between separation and subsequent lack of confidence in the adolescent. Traumatic separation correlated with aggressive traits. Childhood neuroticism was found in those separated at an early age, and inferiority feelings in those separated in the 18 months–6 year groups. Those separated at 18 months–3 years tended to have a lower I.Q. than the rest.

III. TRAUMATIC EXPERIENCES IN CHILDHOOD

It was hypothesized that traumatic experiences other than separation might equally be of importance in the development of subsequent personality traits and psychiatric disturbance. The more of these types of experiences the child had, the more likely he would be to develop trouble later.

A simple yes–no application of this concept established initially that childhood trauma was related to the patient group significantly more often than to controls.

Childhood neurosis, which was conveniently also considered in this section, did not correlate with adolescent breakdown significantly. It did however show a significant positive correlation with a family history of mental illness, inadequate mothering, a poor mother–adolescent relationship and an 'abnormal early history'. This latter included separation and traumatic experiences.

An attempt to relate personality traits to childhood trauma produced positive results for ability to mix, the patients being significantly poorer in this respect, but this did not relate to a separation experience, or to traumatic experiences specifically. Specific phobias however, in the shape of fears of the dark did correlate with separation at the 0.01 level. There was no correlation between phobias and the presence of adolescent breakdown.

From the correlation matrix it is seen that aggressiveness as a trait relates to an abnormal early history, a bad separation experience and a bad father relationship.

Obsessionality related only to the later separation experiences.

Anxiety correlated with poor parental relationships, and an abnormal early history, this latter however not quite reaching statistical significance.

Moodiness related to poor early parental relationships.

Looking at this in the reverse way it is found that abnormal early history correlates with adolescent breakdown at the 5 per cent level of significance. It also correlates with personality disorder, aggressive personality, a poor self-rating by the adolescent, and an inability to achieve adequate close relationships.

In particular poor mother–child relationships tended to occur more commonly in the patient group and correlated with personality disorder, mood disturbance, anxiety, a poor patient self-rating, and with the presence of childhood neurosis.

A poor father–child relationship also occurred more commonly in the patient group, and correlated with personality disorder, moodiness, and poor self-rating. The sex of the patient did not appear significant in this study in this respect.

Thus it was established that the presence of trauma and other abnormalities in the early history did appear to relate to certain aspects of the adolescent's personality and functioning, and this could be shown even by a simple quantitative and relatively crude measure. It is the interaction of all these variables that cannot be disentangled, at any rate without very much more elaborate and sophisticated techniques. The moral nevertheless would appear to be that to keep these episodes in a child's life to a minimum is the best way to safeguard him from this aspect of his subsequent problems in adolescence.

The hypothesis that traumatic situations in childhood in general can be related to subsequent personality traits and disabilities was thus proved in those aspects which have been delineated above.

IV. THE CONCEPT OF TOTAL ADEQUATE RELATIONSHIPS

It was hypothesized that a poor ability to maintain empathetic relationships would be found in the patient group, and the poorer these were, the worse the probable outcome. To test this a simple quantitative scale was initially used, the T.A.R. scale.

It was established that the patient group showed a significantly poorer score on the T.A.R. scale than did the controls ($P = 0.02$). When these results were analysed however, by diagnosis, it was found that it was the personality disorders, and the schizophrenics chiefly who showed the low scores. However the scatter was such as to make this measure less valuable in an individual case.

The ability to establish empathetic relationships did not show a significant correlation with separation experience but did show significance if the total sum of 'abnormal early history' was taken, suggesting that it is the summation of childhood trauma rather than any individual item which relates to later breakdown.

V. RELATIONSHIP THERAPY

It was hoped to establish that a type of psychotherapy aimed purely at establishing an empathetic relationship with the patient, with mutual trust and sympathy, but without the requirement of analytical interpretation, would show a significant improvement in prognosis in some cases.

These personality disorders treated with relationship therapy improved in terms of personal relationships and personality adjustment. The ones who did not receive this kind of therapy did not show this improvement.

Other diagnostic groups showed no correlation between relationship therapy and degree of improvement. The significance of the results was not apparent therefore if the whole 50 patients were considered, but only in the diagnostic category of adolescent personality disorder.

Those patients with a good initial T.A.R. score fared better in terms of re-admissions but this is probably because schizophrenics showed a poor T.A.R. and a high re-admission rating, thus weighting the correlation to a bias in this direction.

The final T.A.R. score showed a positive correlation with a good prognosis and lack of residual symptoms. These patients also had a better opinion of themselves and a high level of self-confidence.

Those with low I.Q. were less likely to receive relationship therapy. Those separated at 18 months–3 years appeared more likely to receive relationship therapy. There is no obvious reason for this latter finding except that personality disorders tended to have had separations more commonly at this age.

VI. PROGNOSTIC INDICATORS

A positive family history, a poor T.A.R. score and an abnormal early history all appeared more frequently in adolescents who developed psychiatric disturbance. These adolescents had a poor self-opinion, had had a poor parent–child relationship in earlier years, and had more commonly been subjected to a separation experience. The longer the separation, and its occurrence in the 18 months–3 years age group made them particularly vulnerable. These features therefore should be viewed as factors which may suggest a tendency of that adolescent subsequently to suffer breakdown.

Rating scales designed to quantify aspects of psychopathology and early history all highlight these distinguishing features. The patient group had less satisfactory mothering. Previous personality was assessed by doctor, parent, and patient also as being less well adjusted than in the controls. In other words the parents had recognized early in many cases that all was not well. Mutual understanding between parent and child is again markedly poorer in the patient. This latter particular rating scale proved to be most reliable in distinguishing patient from control.

The presence of psychotic illness led to a poor prognostic estimate, as did the presence of a suicide attempt, and anxiety and aggressiveness in the personality.

A study of the two year follow-up results in the patient group provided a final prognosis and compared this with the indicators considered above.

Bad mothering was shown to correlate with a lowering of I.Q. at the 1 per cent level of significance. These patients were less able to form an empathetic relationship, and had a worse prognosis. I.Q. also showed a significant correlation with separation at the 18 months–3 years age group.

Those patients with mood disorder and thought disorder had a poor prognosis in terms of re-admission and residual symptoms. Patients with monosymptomatic phobias did well. A positive family history showed a poor prognosis. Bad mothering militated against a good outcome.

In terms of the mental age of separation those separated at M.A. 18 months–3 years had a higher rate of re-admission. Those with a good T.A.R.(1) score had fewer re-admissions. The T.A.R.(2) score correlated positively with a good prognosis, a lack of residual symptoms, and a good patient's opinion of himself.

The patient's final opinion of himself correlated with a good T.A.R.(2) score, with absence of a separation experience, and with a good early mother relationship.

Thus in terms of good prognosis, the ability to relate empathetically to others, the absence of separation, and a good mother–child relationship, appear to be factors of significant importance. A good previous personality is helpful, as is absence of psychotic features.

Bad mothering and separation at a critical age may also lower I.Q., and this in turn leads to poorer prognosis.

In those in whom good T.A.R. scores are achieved in the follow-up period, prognosis is improved. This then is the profile which one may expect to find in the good result case.

VII. CONCLUSIONS

It has been established that separation experiences are commoner in patient than control groups, and that abnormal early histories, including a variety of traumas, quantitatively appear more commonly in patients than in controls.

Patients are shown to have a poorer T.A.R. score than controls, and a profile representative of the poor prognosis group can be devised.

Diagnostic formulations are difficult, and syndromes not clearly defined in the early stages of the illness. Using however the broad categories of adolescent personality disorder, psychosis, and anxiety states generally, and referring to the final diagnostic assessment, it is shown that nearly a half of the patients fall into the personality disorder group. Psychotic patients showed, as one might expect, a positive family history, poor relationships, and a poor prognosis.

Anxiety states by and large were easily dealt with and had a good prognosis. These two latter groups presented relatively less of a problem.

The personality disorder however merited further consideration. This group also had a poor T.A.R. score though perhaps for different reasons. There was a high incidence of separation experience. Suicide attempts were common, as was the presence of aggressiveness, and moodiness. The parental relationships, in particular mother–child relationships, had been poor.

In view of the fact that it was in the personality disorders only that relationship therapy seemed to be important, and an absence of it detrimental in terms of prognosis, and that the inability to form empathetic relationships appeared to be related to a high A.E.H. score, it would seem important that in this type of case relationship therapy should be attempted.

With regard to the apparent lowering of I.Q. in those adolescents separated in the 18 months–3-year-old period, it would seem important to attempt to avoid this by prophylactic measures designed to abolish or lower separation anxieties.

In those patients who showed a good outcome, the T.A.R.(2) score reflected the improvement in their ability to relate.

The problem of rating scales is a vexed one, depending partly on personal preferences, but particularly on the validity of the scales used. In this study, the rating scales have reflected the tendencies observed and have proved useful quantitative measures, simple to apply, and providing a degree of objectivity impossible with merely the personal after-impression from a clinical interview. They should not be regarded as serving any purpose beyond this. They exist merely to make clear the trends in the history, and to make comparisons possible between the patients and controls in a meaningful quantitative manner. They claim no validity beyond this.

What then is the message that these studies should leave with us? It is this:

It has been possible to identify certain children at risk and it has been noted that many of the adolescents seen in the series quoted had been identified by parents and other responsible people as being potential problems from an early age. It would seem much more logical in our society that the maximum endeavour should be put into prevention of these problems at a much earlier age by giving help to the children and their families, preferably before the child completes its formative years. The place in which this might first be initiated could well be at the pre-school play group or nursery stage, where trained staff in adequate numbers might be available, as is done in some parts of the United States, to advise and counsel where there appears to be a need.

Secondly, there should be some training given to mothers-to-be and indeed fathers-to-be on those facts which are fairly positively identified concerning the problems which can arise in the early care of children. This subject should be given much more emphasis, preferably before school-leaving age and in training courses for teachers so that important items can be put across before it is too late.

Thirdly, the identification of those adolescents who do come to treatment, and in particular those who are likely to benefit from relationship therapy, should be made as part of an initial assessment procedure. Strenuous efforts should be made for continuity of care in this respect, once those adolescent personality disorders who should respond to such treatment have come to the therapist's attention. It has been shown that fairly simple procedures can be used to screen and identify the type of case with which we should be concerned.

Much of this information and the discussion in this book is by no means new. Bowlby was reporting to the World Health Organization over fifteen years ago, and yet those concerned with the organization of help of this kind for children remain under-staffed, and the availability of units for adolescents remains well below that which is required.

Finally it must be apparent that parents should think much more carefully before they create a separation experience for their child.

That society is making a rod for its own back is suggested by the results of the work quoted concerning the rearing of apes, and is apparent in human society if one cares to look. The deflection of financial resources into this group of problems would pay immense dividends for the future and should, if nothing else, diminish considerably the burden to the community which these problems would otherwise impose.

APPENDICES

1. TABLES OF QUESTIONNAIRES

The pattern followed in devising the questionnaires has been in general on the lines of that described in *The Psychiatric Dilemma of Adolescence* by James F. Masterson and is detailed in full in the appendices of that book, pp. 163–206. Symptom pattern groupings were considered under headings broadly as set out in Table 16, Appendix A, p. 165 of the above reference, namely .

(*a*) Thinking disorder
(*b*) Anxiety patterns
(*c*) Conversion symptoms
(*d*) Phobic pattern
(*e*) Obsessive-compulsive pattern
(*f*) Depressive pattern
(*g*) Hypochondriacal pattern
(*h*) Psychosomatic
(*i*) Behaviour disturbance
(*j*) Intellectual functioning.

At the initial and follow-up interviews consideration was given to: (*i*) symptomatology, (*ii*) social adjustment, (*iii*) family relationships, (*iv*) situation.

In addition the patient was asked to fill in a questionnaire concerning aspects of his personality generally on the lines set out in pp. 199–206 of Masterson's book.

The parents were required to answer fully at interview details of the relevant early history, particularly as it related to separation and this was set out in questionnaire form.

At follow-up in addition to an interview, a formal questionnaire was obtained, to get answers to set standardized questions. This plus a personal letter was all that could be obtained from those patients whom it was not possible to interview personally.

2. COMPUTER PROGRAMMING DETAILS

The computer used was that of the University of Newcastle upon Tyne Computing Laboratory. This is a KDF9 computer using Whetstone Algol (WALGOL). A program suitable for psychiatric statistical research was in use at the Department of Psychological Medicine, Newcastle upon Tyne University Medical School and this program would give a regression analysis, producing a correlation matrix for a variable number of factors.

The method of determining correlation coefficients in use in this program is that of the 'product-moment' method.

The rank-difference correlation method is best used for small numbers (15–30) and is simpler. The product-moment method is however more accurate since it takes into account the absolute size of the measures and not merely rank order. Rank order was in this study often not appropriate, and the numbers ran to 100 maximum.

A list is now given of the items fed into the computer.

Matrix A

This included 100 individuals and concerned initial assessment and comparisons of previous history and personality between patient and control. There were 38 items here listed and explained.

1.	Sex	male—female
2.	Patient/control	patient—control
3.	Diagnosis schizophrenia	present—absent
4.	Diagnosis depressive	present—absent
5.	Diagnosis anxiety	present—absent
6.	Diagnosis personality disorder	present—absent
7.	Age of onset	early—late onset
8.	Symptom—affective	present—absent
9.	Symptom—suicide attempt	present—absent
10.	Symptom—aggression	present—absent
11.	Symptom—obsessional	present—absent
12.	Symptom—ideas of reference	present—absent
13.	Symptom—anxiety	present—absent
14.	Symptom—phobic	present—absent
15.	Symptom—moodiness	present—absent
**25.*	Symptom—delusional	present—absent
26.	Symptom—manneristic	present—absent

16.	Sibling order	only child—large family
17.	Family history	present—none
18.	Childhood neurotic features	present—absent
19.	Child–parent relationships	good—poor
20.	Unsatisfactory mother scale	good mother—bad mother
21.	Total adequate relationships	few—many
22.	Abnormal early history	present—absent
23.	Patient's adjustment rating	poor adjustment—good adjustment
24.	Mother–child empathy	low—high
*27.	Father–child relationship	good—bad
28.	Separation experience	present—absent
29.	'Substitute parent' during separation	satisfactory—unsatisfactory
30.	Immediate after-effect of separation	no problems—problems
31.	Length of separation	short—long
32.	Age of separation 6 months	present—none
33.	Age of separation 6 months to 1 year	present—none
34.	Age of separation 1 year to 18 months	present—none
35.	Age of separation 18 months to 3 years	present—none
36.	Age of separation 3 years to 4 years	present—none
37.	Age of separation 4 years	present—none
38.	Initial prognostic assessment (i.e. on discharge)	good—bad

The results of this matrix are presented in Appendix 3A.

Matrix B

This included 50 patients and was concerned with the two year follow-up. Items of early history and separation were compared with follow-up assessment. Twenty-three items were included as follows:

1.	I.Q.	low—high
2.	Symptom—mood disorder (at initial assessment)	present—absent
3.	Symptom—obsessional	present—absent
4.	Symptom—anxiety	present—absent

5. Symptom—phobic	present—absent
6. Symptom—aggression	present—absent
**18.* Symptom—delusional	present—absent
7. Childhood neurosis	present—absent
8. Unsatisfactory mother scale	good mother—bad mother
9. Total adequate relationships	Few—many
10. Abnormal early history	present—none
19. Length of separation	short—long
20. Mental age of separation 18 months	present—none
21. Mental age of separation 18 months to 3 years	present—none
22. Mental age of separation 3 years	present—none
11. Transference relationship in therapy	present—absent
12. Follow-up after discharge	yes—no
13. Residual symptoms at 2 year assessment	yes—no
14. Final prognosis	good—bad
15. Re-admissions	none—many
16. Final patient's self-rating	good—poor
17. Final total adequate relationships score	few—many
23. Final adjustment rating	good—poor

The results of this matrix are presented in Appendix 3B.

* The numbers refer to the numbers on p. 109–111 but they have been put here in a more rational order appropriate to the assessment questionnaire.

3. CORRELATION MATRICES

CORRLN. COEFFS

VAR	1	2	3	4	5	6	7	8	9	10	11	12	13	14
1	1.0000													
2	0.0629	1.0000												
3	0.0155	0.2949	1.000											
4	-0.0061	0.1759	-0.0519	1.0000										
5	0.0785	0.5620	-0.0794	-0.0988	1.0000									
6	-0.0354	0.5311	-0.1566	0.0481	-0.0158	1.0000								
7	-0.0885	-0.9507	-0.2529	-0.1963	0.5719	-0.4858	1.0000							
8	0.0175	0.7500	0.0860	0.2345	0.4566	0.4567	-0.6894	1.0000						
9	0.0349	0.3333	0.0246	-0.0586	0.0468	0.3862	-0.2933	0.3750	1.0000					
10	0.0927	0.2949	0.1848	-0.0519	0.0069	0.1993	-0.2638	0.1628	0.2703	1.0000				
11	-0.1487	0.4364	0.0724	0.0831	0.3934	0.0975	-0.3421	0.3546	-0.0546	0.0724	1.0000			
12	0.0623	0.3145	0.2937	0.3544	0.0131	0.1704	-0.3097	0.2009	0.1281	0.2937	0.0534	1.0000		
13	-0.0090	0.6002	0.1928	0.0050	0.3172	0.3602	-0.5377	0.4234	0.0572	0.1138	0.4023	0.1588	1.0000	
14	0.0703	-0.2643	-0.2458	-0.1466	-0.0400	-0.1482	0.2583	-0.2440	-0.1423	-0.2458	0.0244	-0.1911	-0.0052	1.0000
15	0.0229	0.4364	-0.0282	0.0831	0.2018	0.2950	-0.4468	0.5251	0.4001	0.2735	0.1815	0.1487	0.3438	-0.0865
16	0.1517	-0.0629	-0.1146	-0.0058	-0.0606	-0.0030	0.0866	-0.0996	0.0539	0.1173	0.0020	-0.0575	0.0223	0.0791
17	-0.0048	0.4104	0.4135	0.0294	0.2007	0.1255	-0.4058	0.2679	0.1064	0.2454	0.0522	0.1322	0.1799	-0.1233
18	-0.0279	0.1435	0.1421	-0.0204	-0.1613	0.2188	-0.1297	0.0837	0.0068	0.1421	-0.0693	-0.0365	0.1547	-0.0413
19	-0.0111	0.0303	0.0959	0.0683	-0.1360	0.0175	-0.0446	0.1179	-0.0555	0.1238	-0.0644	0.1750	0.0285	-0.1172
20	0.0274	-0.1454	-0.1400	0.0585	-0.0399	-0.0066	0.1052	-0.0028	-0.0452	-0.1043	-0.0354	0.0369	-0.1699	-0.0116
21	0.0537	0.3329	0.1935	0.0450	0.0839	0.2751	-0.3890	0.2187	0.1280	0.2171	0.0943	0.1700	0.0247	-0.0469
22	0.0409	0.2170	0.1536	0.0280	-0.1646	0.2242	-0.1555	0.0741	0.1013	0.2335	0.0497	-0.1016	0.1712	-0.0291
23	-0.1034	0.4646	0.3774	0.1773	-0.0443	0.4042	-0.3815	0.3824	0.1005	0.2271	0.0694	0.3740	0.3886	-0.0767
24	0.2233	0.3677	0.1504	0.0744	0.0429	0.3922	-0.3327	0.3029	0.1642	0.1759	0.0333	0.1816	0.3647	-0.1127
25	0.1700	0.2949	0.5924	0.1642	0.0069	-0.0676	-0.2529	0.1628	-0.0983	0.0489	0.1729	0.2937	0.1138	-0.0959
26	0.0771	0.3516	0.4854	0.1255	0.1018	-0.0447	-0.2980	0.0692	-0.1172	0.0141	0.1081	0.2245	0.1014	-0.0981
27	0.0374	-0.3118	-0.1445	-0.1514	-0.0668	-0.2602	0.2291	-0.2283	-0.0891	-0.2266	-0.1531	-0.1930	-0.2406	0.0670
28	-0.0213	0.2478	0.1528	0.1571	0.0274	0.2208	-0.1800	0.1539	-0.0526	0.0697	0.0418	0.2810	0.0657	-0.0490
29	-0.0623	-0.1747	-0.4225	0.0553	0.0949	-0.0017	0.1446	0.0175	0.1048	-0.2937	-0.0534	-0.2674	-0.0090	0.1201
30	-0.0349	-0.1333	-0.2703	0.0586	0.0312	0.0161	0.0964	-0.0278	-0.0000	-0.2703	-0.0364	-0.1281	0.0143	0.0746
31	-0.0150	-0.2380	-0.2842	-0.0474	0.0156	0.1528	0.1452	-0.1279	-0.0238	-0.1526	-0.0636	-0.2511	-0.0490	0.0493
32	-0.0061	0.0586	0.1642	-0.0309	-0.0988	0.0481	0.0114	-0.0098	-0.0586	0.1642	0.0831	0.1495	0.1307	-0.0274
33	0.1202	-0.0459	-0.0677	-0.0403	-0.0215	0.0111	0.0284	0.0191	0.0765	0.1015	-0.1001	-0.0721	-0.1574	0.0886
34	-0.1290	-0.0586	-0.0519	-0.0309	-0.0988	0.0481	0.0633	-0.0098	-0.0586	-0.0519	0.0831	-0.0553	0.0050	-0.0274
35	-0.0966	0.2676	0.1052	0.1063	0.1309	0.2254	-0.1856	-0.1437	-0.0297	-0.0044	0.0746	0.1901	0.1173	-0.1409
36	-0.0428	0.1021	0.3160	0.2633	-0.1147	0.0148	-0.0621	0.0595	-0.0680	0.1279	0.0501	0.4708	-0.0306	-0.0664
37	-0.0737	0.1005	0.3408	-0.0177	-0.0565	-0.0534	0.0659	0.1340	-0.0335	0.3408	0.2303	0.3196	0.1465	-0.0838
38	0.0734	-0.4201	-0.4955	-0.0903	-0.0262	-0.1825	0.3613	-0.2684	-0.2334	-0.3923	-0.1222	-0.2593	-0.3122	0.2932

Matrix A—variables 1–14

VAR	15	16	17	18	19	20	21	22	23	24	25	26	27	28
15	1.0000													
16	0.0020	1.0000												
17	-0.0721	-0.0537	1.0000											
18	0.0425	0.1487	0.2739	1.0000										
19	0.2039	-0.0125	-0.1435	-0.0617	1.0000									
20	0.0174	0.0359	-0.2262	-0.2505	0.1086	1.0000								
21	0.2340	-0.0817	0.1518	0.0341	0.1540	-0.1669	1.0000							
22	0.1681	0.1927	0.2097	0.3941	-0.0053	-0.5097	0.2556	1.0000						
23	0.2695	-0.0836	0.1825	0.1710	0.4978	-0.1348	0.4185	0.2798	1.0000					
24	0.3171	0.1158	0.0927	0.2104	0.1838	-0.0041	0.1714	0.2538	0.4254	1.0000				
25	-0.1287	-0.1477	0.4135	-0.0091	0.0402	-0.0507	0.0755	0.1536	0.1971	0.2015	1.0000			
26	0.0209	-0.0164	0.3017	-0.0190	-0.1939	-0.2444	0.1923	0.2178	0.2415	0.0157	0.4854	1.0000		
27	-0.2138	-0.0829	-0.0366	-0.1406	-0.1860	0.1127	-0.3736	-0.2764	-0.5257	-0.4493	-0.1445	-0.2078	1.0000	
28	-0.0197	0.1419	0.2044	0.2064	0.1387	-0.1578	0.1125	0.3411	0.2826	0.1324	0.3188	0.3621	-0.1726	1.0000
29	-0.0534	-0.1781	-0.1322	-0.1784	-0.0957	0.1155	-0.1253	-0.4291	-0.2316	-0.1331	-0.4225	-0.3362	0.1930	-0.5171
30	-0.0364	-0.1887	-0.1064	-0.1435	0.0807	0.1744	-0.0854	-0.4629	-0.1549	-0.0948	-0.2703	-0.2024	0.1633	-0.5481
31	-0.0636	-0.1360	-0.1508	-0.1181	0.1267	0.2543	-0.1493	-0.4275	-0.3402	-0.1555	-0.2842	-0.3863	0.1770	-0.8608
32	0.0831	0.1523	-0.1042	0.2199	0.0683	-0.0267	0.1201	0.0280	0.1773	0.1558	-0.0519	-0.0618	-0.1514	0.2892
33	-0.1001	0.1093	0.0732	0.0988	-0.1423	-0.1089	0.0587	0.1692	-0.0430	-0.0939	-0.0677	-0.0807	0.0409	0.3772
34	-0.0768	0.0732	0.0294	0.0998	-0.0204	0.0585	-0.1801	-0.0992	-0.0616	0.0744	0.1642	-0.0618	0.1097	0.2892
35	-0.0065	0.0184	0.1776	-0.0043	-0.1723	-0.1547	0.0800	0.3626	0.2038	0.0811	0.3244	0.4343	-0.1563	0.6356
36	-0.0891	-0.0679	0.2280	0.1507	0.1050	-0.1464	-0.0131	0.1063	0.3028	0.0156	0.3160	0.2544	-0.1000	0.3356
37	-0.0439	-0.0334	0.1696	-0.0804	0.0897	-0.1938	-0.1029	0.1614	0.2925	-0.0272	0.3408	0.2859	-0.1612	0.1653
38	-0.1222	-0.0239	-0.3895	-0.1809	-0.2479	-0.0312	-0.1255	-0.1884	-0.5148	-0.3138	-0.2890	-0.1208	0.1746	-0.1230

VAR	29	30	31	32	33	34	35	36	37	38
29	1.0000									
30	0.8270	1.0000								
31	0.5421	0.6584	1.0000							
32	-0.1495	-0.1368	-0.3264	1.0000						
33	-0.0882	-0.3824	-0.4258	-0.0403	1.0000					
34	0.0553	0.0586	-0.1869	0.3127	-0.0403	1.0000				
35	-0.3979	-0.3667	-0.5406	-0.0680	-0.0887	-0.0680	1.0000			
36	-0.4708	-0.2722	-0.2574	-0.0359	-0.0468	-0.0359	0.0728	1.0000		
37	-0.3196	-0.3015	-0.3061	-0.0177	-0.0231	-0.0177	0.2600	0.4924	1.0000	
38	0.1615	0.1400	0.1799	-0.0903	0.0964	-0.0903	-0.1707	-0.0572	-0.2392	1.0000

Matrix A—variables 15–38

CORRLN. COEFFS

VAR	1	2	3	4	5	6	7	8	9	10	11	12	13	14
1	1.0000													
2	-0.0022	1.0000												
3	-0.1189	0.0458	1.0000											
4	0.0909	-0.0546	0.2100	1.0000										
5	-0.1080	-0.1071	0.2406	0.3273	1.0000									
6	0.2204	-0.0754	-0.1762	-0.0987	-0.1938	1.0000								
7	0.0263	-0.0500	-0.2030	0.0983	-0.0393	0.2328	1.0000							
8	-0.3836	0.2059	0.0399	-0.0789	-0.1081	-0.2826	-0.2229	1.0000						
9	-0.0808	-0.0668	-0.0700	-0.2649	-0.1120	0.0544	0.0854	-0.1297	1.0000					
10	0.1180	-0.1679	-0.0627	0.0157	-0.0891	0.1612	0.3642	-0.4604	0.2028	1.0000				
11	-0.4194	-0.1273	0.1400	0.0833	-0.0546	-0.2303	-0.0164	0.1148	-0.0355	-0.0157	1.0000			
12	-0.0977	-0.1655	-0.0507	0.1896	0.0715	0.0408	0.2389	0.1217	-0.1616	-0.1526	0.3275	1.0000		
13	-0.1037	-0.2548	-0.0898	0.2303	-0.1041	0.1883	0.1520	0.0538	-0.0129	0.0062	0.0987	0.3810	1.0000	
14	-0.0351	0.0778	0.0748	-0.0891	0.3110	-0.2989	-0.1839	-0.1304	0.0029	-0.1343	0.0000	-0.1935	-0.6506	1.0000
15	0.0070	0.0699	0.2207	0.0766	0.1579	0.0234	0.0212	-0.1651	-0.3367	-0.1665	-0.2157	-0.3544	-01072	-0.3311
16	0.0322	-0.0650	0.0156	-0.0186	0.1665	-0.0257	0.0897	-0.2837	-0.0177	0.1473	0.0186	-0.0404	-0.3931	0.5074
17	0.1151	-0.0039	0.2100	0.2035	0.2935	0.0803	-0.1278	-0.0431	-0.1053	-0.0850	-0.0708	-0.1254	-0.3999	0.4115
18	0.1269	-0.0923	0.0515	-0.0891	-0.0292	0.3825	-0.0744	-0.0105	-0.0263	0.1175	-0.1336	0.3132	0.1627	-0.1905
19	0.1415	0.1057	0.0404	0.1503	-0.0601	-0.0561	-0.1535	0.2075	-0.1637	-0.4265	-0.2339	-0.0665	-0.0561	0.1205
20	-0.0259	-0.0439	0.0106	-0.0754	0.0439	0.1686	0.2766	-0.1915	0.1013	0.3361	-0.0503	0.0052	0.1686	-0.2955
21	-0.2444	0.0292	-0.1824	-0.0891	-0.0292	0.0528	-0.0744	0.0854	-0.0810	0.0126	0.3118	0.0829	0.0528	0.0476
22	-0.1879	-0.1445	0.1138	-0.0602	0.1445	-0.1129	0.1716	0.0091	0.1795	0.0794	0.0602	0.2117	-0.1129	0.1930
23	-0.0775	0.1558	0.0456	-0.0994	0.1893	-0.1195	-0.0719	-0.0191	-0.0663	-0.1243	-0.0361	-0.1878	-0.6546	0.7294

VAR	15	16	17	18	19	20	21	22	23
15	1.0000								
16	0.1858	1.0000							
17	0.1600	0.3528	1.0000						
18	-0.3013	0.1343	0.2223	1.0000					
19	0.3812	-0.2827	0.0262	-0.2813	1.0000				
20	-0.1763	0.2189	0.0213	0.3425	-0.6472	1.0000			
21	-0.2548	0.0099	0.0449	-0.0417	-0.3929	-0.1612	1.0000		
22	-0.1408	0.1748	-0.0096	0.2735	-0.1900	-0.1089	-0.1287	1.0000	
23	0.3430	0.6167	0.5838	-0.0314	0.0485	-0.1117	0.0894	0.1012	1.0000

Matrix B—all variables

REFERENCES

Ahnsjö, S. (1941). *Acta paediat., Stockh.* **28,** 3, 1. In *Maternal Care and Mental Health*, p. 162. By J. Bowlby. W.H.O. Geneva

Aichhorn, A. (1935). Wayward youth. New York; Viking

Ainsworth, M. D. (1962). 'Deprivation of maternal care—a re-assessment of its effects.' p. 97. Public Health paper, no. 14. W.H.O. Geneva

— and Bowlby, J. (1954). 'Research strategy in the study of mother–child separation'. *Courrier*, **4,** No. 3, 2

Albrecht, H. (1966). 'The present situation of child and juvenile psychiatry in W. Germany.' *Acta Paedopsychiat., (Basel)* **33,** 258

Am. J. Psychiat. (1967). Editorial. **123,** 1031

Annesley, P. T. (1961). 'Psychiatric illness in adolescence. Its presentation and prognosis.' *J. ment. Sci.* **107,** 268

Armstrong, C. R. (1932). 660 runaway boys. Why boys desert from their homes. Boston, Mass; Humphries

Aubry, J. (1955). La carence de soins maternals. Paris; Centre International de l'Enfance

Bakwin, H. (1942). 'Loneliness in infants.' *Am. J. Dis. Child.* **63,** 30

— (1949). 'Emotional deprivation in infants.' *J. Pediat.* **35,** 512

Balser, B. H. and Masterson, J. F. (1959). 'Suicide in adolescents.' *Am. J. Psychiat.* **116,** 400

Barry, H. (1949). 'Significance of maternal bereavement before age of eight in psychiatric patients.' *Archs Neurol. Psychiat., Chicago* **62,** 630

Becker, W. C. (1964). 'Consequences of different kinds of parental discipline.' In *Review of Child Development Research*, Vol. 1. New York; Russell Sage Foundation

Bender, L. (1947). 'Psychopathic behaviour disorders in children.' In *Handbook of Correctional Psychology*, p. 360. Ed. by R. M. Lindner and R. V. Seligan, New York; Philosophical Library

Beres, D. and Obers, S. J. (1950). 'The effects of extreme deprivation in infancy on psychic structure in adolescence: a study in age development.' In *Psychoanalytic Study of the Child*, Vol. 5, p. 212. New York; International Universities Press

Bernfeld, S. (1923). 'Uber eine typische Form des Männlichen Pubertät.' *Imago* 9. In *The psychiatric dilemma of adolescence*, p. 7. By J. F. Masterson. London; J. & A. Churchill Ltd.

Blau, A. (1952). 'In support of Freud's Syndrome of Actual Anxiety Neurosis.' *Int. J. Psycho-Analysis* **33,** 363

Bovet, L. (1951). 'Psychiatric aspects of juvenile delinquency.' Monograph series. No. 1. W.H.O. Geneva

Bowlby, J. (1940). 'The influence of early environment in the development of neuroses and neurotic character.' *Int. J. Psycho-Analysis* **21,** 154

— (1946). 44 juvenile thieves: their characters and home life. London; Bailliere, Tyndall & Cox

— (1951). 'Maternal Care and Mental Health.' W.H.O. Geneva

— Ainsworth, M., Boston, M. and Rosenbluth, D. (1956). 'The effects of mother–child separation: A follow-up study.' *Br. J. med. Psychol.* **29,** 211

Boyd, P. R. (1967). Proceedings of N.A.M.H. Annual Conference. 1967

Braceland, J. F. (1937). 'Behaviour problems, definition and scope.' *Med. J. Penn.* **41,** 180

Br. med. J. (1960). Leading Article. 'Adolescence.' **2,** 281

Burlingham, D. and Freud, A. (1942). Annual report of a residential war nursery. London; Allen & Unwin

— — (1942). Young children in wartime. London; Allen & Unwin

Burr, C. W. (1905). 'Insanity at puberty.' *J. Am. med. Ass.* **45,** 36

Burt, C. (1929). The young delinquent. London; Appleton

Caldwell, B. M. (1964). 'The effects of infant care.' In *Review of Child Development Research*, Vol. 1. New York; Russell Sage Foundation

Capes, M., Gould, E. and Townsend, M. (1971). Stress in youth. Nuffield Provincial Hospitals Trust, London; Oxford University Press

Caplan, M. G. and Douglas, V. I. (1969). 'Incidence of parental loss in children with depressed mood.' *J. Child Psychol. Psychiat.* **10,** 225

Carter, A. B. (1942). 'Prognostic factors in psychosis in adolescence.' *J. ment. Sci.* **88,** 31

Clouston, T. S. (1891). Neuroses of development. Edinburgh; Oliver and Boyd

Cohen, A. (1956). Delinquent boys. London, Routledge & Kegan Paul

Corner, G. W. (1944). Ourselves unborn. In *Maternal Care and Mental Health*, p. 54. By J. Bowlby. W.H.O. Geneva

Cowan, E. A. and Stout, E. (1939). 'A comparative study of adjustment made by foster children after complete–partial breaks in continuity of home environment.' *Am. J. Orthopsychiat.* **9,** 330

Curran, F. J. (1939). 'Organization of a ward for adolescents in the Bellevue psychopathic hospital.' *Am. J. Psychiat.* **5,** 1365

Daily, J. M. (1959). 'School characteristics of male adolescents who later became schizophrenic.' *Proceedings of N.A.M.H. annual conference*, p. 712

Dawson, W. S. (1935). 'Psychoses in adolescence.' *Br. med. J.* **2,** 651

Donelli, A., Faienza, C. and Moretti, M. (1965). 'Study of effect of lack of maternal care in adolescents.' *Lattante* **36,** 291

Douglas, J. W. B. (1964). The home and the school. London; MacGibbon & Kee

— (1970). 'Broken families and child behaviour.' *Jnl. R. Coll. Physicians Lond.* **4,** (3), 203

Douglas, J. W. B. and Blomfield, J. M. (1958). Children under five. London; Allen & Unwin

— Ross, J. M. and Simpson, H. R. (1968). All our futures. A longitudinal study of secondary education. London; Peter Davies

Earle, A. M. and Earle, B. V. (1961). 'Early maternal deprivation and later psychiatric illness.' *Am. J. Orthopsychiat.* **31,** 181

Engel, M. (1959). 'The stability of the self concept in adolescence.' *J. abnorm. Psychol.* **58,** 211

Erikson, E. H. (1959). 'Identity and the life cycle.' *Psychol. Issues* **1,** 1

Freud, A. (1946). Psychoanalytic treatment of children (1927). London; Imago Publishing Co.

— (1958). 'Adolescence.' In *Psychoanalytic Study of the Child.* Vol. 13. p. 255. New York; International University Press

Freud, S. (1953). Three essays on the theory of sexuality. Vol. 7. London; Hogarth.

Gesell, A. and Amatruda, C. (1947). 'Developmental diagnosis: normal and abnormal child development.' In *Clinical methods and paediatric applications.* 2nd ed. New York; Hoeber

Gibbens, T. C. N. (1961). 'Psychiatric aspects of delinquency.' Public Health paper no. 5. W.H.O. Geneva

Gibson, H. B. (1969). 'Early delinquency in relation to broken homes.' *J. Child Psychol. Psychiat.* **12,** 195

Gillespie, R. D. and Lay, R. A. Q. (1936). 'Prognosis of psychological disturbances in adolescents and school children.' *Lancet* **1,** 1129

Glueck, S. and Glueck, E. T. (1934). One thousand juvenile delinquents. Cambridge, Massachussetts; Harvard University Press

Goldfarb, W. (1943). 'Effects of early institutional care on adolescent personality.' *J. exp. Educ.* **12,** 106

— (1943). 'Infant rearing and problem behaviour (1).' *Am. J. Orthopsychiat.* **13,** 249

— (1947). 'Infant rearing and problem behaviour. (2).' *Am. J. Orthopsychiat.* **17,** 449

Gregory, I. (1958). 'Studies of parental deprivation in psychiatric patients.' *Am. J. Psychiat.* **115,** (5), 432

Hall, M. B. (1938). 'Juvenile nervous and mental instability. Study of 1000 cases.' *Lancet* **2,** 272

Harlow, H. F. (1961). 'Mother–infant interactions in monkeys.' Paper delivered at Tavistock Study Group, 1961. London

Hebb, D. O. (1949). The organization of behaviour. New York; Wiley

Henderson, A. S., McCulloch, J. W. and Philip, A. E. (1967). 'Survey of mental illness in adolescence.' *Br. med. J.* **1,** 83

Hewitt, L. E. and Jenkins, R. L. (1946). The fundamental patterns of maladjustment. Springfield, Illinois; Michigan Child Guidance Institute publication

Hill, O. and Price, J. (1967). 'Childhood bereavement and adult depression.' *Br. J. Psychiat.* **113,** 743

Hinde, R. A. and Spencer-Booth, Y. (1970). 'Individual differences in the responses of rhesus monkeys to a period of separation from their mothers.' *J. Child Psychol. Psychiat.* **11,** 159

Howells, J. G. and Layng, J. (1955). 'Separation experiences and mental health.' *Lancet* **2,** 285

Isaacs, S. (1948). 'Children in institutions.' In *Childhood and After. Some essays–clinical studies.* p. 205. London; International University Press

Jackson, K., Winkley, R., Faust, O. A. and Cermak, E. G. (1952). 'Problems of emotional trauma in hospital treatment of children.' *J. Am. med. Ass.* **149,** 1536

Jones, E. (1922). 'Some problems of adolescence.' Papers on psychoanalysis. 5th ed. (1948). London; Bailliere, Tindall & Cox

Kasanin, J. (1931). 'Affective psychoses in children.' *Am. J. Psychiat.* **10,** 897

— and Kaufmann, M. (1929). 'A study of the functional psychoses of childhood.' *Am. J. Psychiat.* **9,** 307

Kraepelin, E. (1896). Psychiatrie. 5th ed. Leipzig; Thieme

Lancet (1964). 'Suicide and suicide attempts in children and adolescents.' Leading article. **2,** 847

Lancet (1967). Crisis at Adolescence. Annotation. **1,** 486

League of Nations (1938). Prostitutes. Their early lives. Geneva

League of Nations (1938). The placing of children in families. Vol. 1, p. 8. Geneva

Levy, D. M. (1937). 'Primary affect hunger.' *Am. J. Psychiat.* **94,** 643

Lewis, H. (1954). Deprived children. (The Mershal experiment). A social and clinical study. London; Oxford University Press

Lidz, R. W. and Lidz, T. (1949). 'Family environment of schizophrenic patients.' *Am. J. Psychiat.* **106,** 332

Lowrey, L. G. (1940). 'Personality distortion and early infant care.' *Am. J. Orthopsychiat.* **10,** 576

McCulloch, J. W., Henderson, A. S. and Philip, A. E. (1966). 'Psychiatric illness in Edinburgh teenagers.' *Scott med. J.* **11,** 277

McGregor, H. G. (1944). 'Physical examination of 2000 cases of neurosis.' *J. Neurol. Psychiat.* **7,** 21

Madow, L. and Hardy, S. E. (1947). 'Incidence and analysis of broken family in background of neurosis.' *Am. J. Orthopsychiat.* **17,** 521

Masterson, J. F. (1956). 'Prognosis in adolescent disorders.' *J. Neurol. ment. Dis.* **124,** 219

— (1958). 'Prognosis in adolescent disorders.' *Am. J. Psychiat.* **114,** 1097

— (1967). 'The symptomatic adolescent five years later.' *Am. J. Psychiat.* **123,** 1338

— (1967). The psychiatric dilemma of adolescence. London; J. & A. Churchill, Ltd

— Tucker, K. and Berk, G. (1963). 'Psychopathology in adolescents—clinical and dynamic characteristics.' *Am. J. Psychiat.* **120,** 357

— and Washbourne, A. (1966). 'The symptomatic adolescent. Psychiatric illness or adolescent turmoil.' *Am. J. Psychiat.* **122,** 1240

Mathis, M. (1964). 'La rôle du père dans l'inadaptation des adolescents.' *Strasbourg med. J.* **15,** 53

Mead, A. M. (1962). 'A cultural anthropologist's approach to maternal deprivation. Deprivation of Maternal Care. A re-assessment of its effects.' p. 45. Public Health paper no. 14. W.H.O. Geneva

Meierhofer, H. (1950). Homeless children. Paris; UNESCO

Menut, G. (1943). La dissociation familiale et les troubles du caractère chez l'enfant. Paris. In *Maternal Care and Mental Health,* p. 12. By J. Bowlby. W.H.O. Geneva

Ministry of Health (1944). Hostels for 'difficult' children. A survey of experience under the evacuation scheme, London

Ministry of Health (1964). In-patient accommodation for mentally ill and seriously maladjusted children and adolescents H.M. (64) 4

Morel, B. A. (1860). Traité des dégénereuse physiques. Paris; Masson

Naess, S. (1959). 'Mother–child separation and delinquency.' *Br. J. Delinq.* **10,** 22

Phillips, L. J. (1953). 'Case history data and prognosis in schizophrenia.' *Nerv. ment. Dis.* **117,** 515

Pickerill, C. and Pickerill, H. P. (1947). 'Plastic surgery clinic for babies, whose mothers reside with their infants.' *Nursing Mirror* August 16th, II–IV

Pitt, R. (1964). 'Patterns of peer interaction during adolescence as prognostic indicators in schizophrenia.' *Am. J. Psychiat.* **120,** 1089

Pitts, F. H., Meyer, J., Brooks, M. and Wincker, G. (1965). *Am. J. Psychiat.* **121,** Suppl. June

Pollock, H. M., Malzberg, B. and Fuller, R. G. (1939). Hereditary and environmental factors in the causation of manic-depressive psychoses and dementia praecox. New York; Utica

Powdermaker, F., Levis, H. T. and Touraine, G. (1937). 'Psychopathology and treatment of delinquent females.' *Am. J. Orthopsychiat.* **7,** 58

Pringle, M. L. K. and Bossio, V. (1960). 'Early prolonged separation and emotional maladjustment.' *J. Child Psychol. Psychiat.* **1,** 37

Prugh, D. G., Staub, E. M., Sands, H. H., Kirschbaun, R. M. and Lenihan, E. A. (1953). 'A study of emotional reactions of children and families to hospitalization and illness.' *Am. J. Orthopsychiat.* **23,** 70

Ribble, M. (1943). The rights of infants. Early psychological Needs and their satisfaction. New York; Columbia University Press

Robertson, J. (1953). 'Some responses of young children to the loss of maternal care.' *Nursing Times* **49,** 382

Robins, L. N. and O'Neal, P. (1958). 'Mortality, morbidity and crime: Problem children 30 years later.' *Am. Sociol. Rev.* **23,** 162

Rutter, M. (1971). 'Parent child separation—Psychological effects on the children.' *J. Child Psychol. Psychiat.* **12,** 233

— (1972). Maternal deprivation reassessed. Harmonsworth, England; Penguin Education

Sands, D. E. (1953). 'A special mental hospital unit for treatment of psychosis and neurosis in juveniles.' *J. ment. Sci.* **414,** 123

Schaffer, H. R. (1958). 'Objective observations of personality development in early infancy.' *Br. J. med. Psychol.* **31,** 174

Schroeder, P. L. (1939). 'Behaviour problems of adolescents.' *Am. J. Dis. Child.* **58,** 168

Spiegel, L. A. (1951). 'A review of contributions to a psychoanalytic theory of adolescence.' In *The Psychoanalytic Study of the Child.* Vol. 6, p. 375. New York; International University Press

Spitz, R. A. and Wolf, K. M. (1946). 'Anaclitic depression: an inquiry into the genesis of psychiatric conditions in early childhood.' In *The Psychoanalytic Study of the Child.* Vol. 2, p. 313. New York; International University Press

Stacey, M., Dearden, R., Pitt, R. and Robinson, D. (1970). Hospitals, children and their families. The report of a pilot study. London; Routledge & Kegan Paul

Stott, D. H. (1956). 'The effects of separation from the mother in early life.' *Lancet* **1,** 624

Sukhereva, G. E. and Kogan, E. I. (1933). 'Prognosis of cases of schizophrenia at puberty.' *Sov. Psikhonevrol.* **6,** 126

Sullivan, H. S. (1956). Clinical studies in psychiatry. New York; W. W. Norton

Teicher, J. D. and Jacobs, J. (1966). 'Adolescents who attempt suicide: preliminary findings.' *Am. J. Psychiat.* **122,** 1248

Toolan, J. M. (1962). 'Suicide and suicidal attempts in children and adolescents.' *Am. J. Psychiat.* **118,** 719

Trasler, G. (1960). In place of parents. London; Routledge & Kegan Paul

Turner, C. H., Davenport, R. K. and Rogers, C. M. (1969). 'The effect of early deprivation on the social behaviour of adolescent chimpanzees.' *Am. J. Psychiat.* **125,** 153

Wardle, C. J. (1961). 'Two generations of broken homes in the genesis of conduct and behaviour disorders in childhood.' *Br. med. J.* **2,** 349

Warren, W. (1949). 'Abnormal behaviour and mental breakdown in adolescence.' *J. ment. Sci.* **95,** 589

— (1965). 'A study of adolescent psychiatric in-patients and the outcome six or more years later.' *J. Child Psychol. Psychiat.* **6,** 1

— and Cameron, K. (1950). 'Reactive psychosis in adolescence.' *J. ment. Sci.* **96,** 403

Wertz, F. J., (1962). 'The fate of behaviour disorders in adolescence.' *Am. J. Orthopsychiat.* **32,** 423

Wilson, H. (1960). 'Psychological and psychiatric disturbances in adolescence.' *Practitioner* **184,** 301

Wittman, M. P. and Huffman, A. V. (1945). 'Comparative study of developmental adjustment and personality characteristics of psychotic pseudoneurotic, delinquent and normally adjusted teenaged youths.' *J. genet Psychol.* **66,** 167

Wooton, B. (1962). 'A social scientist's approach to maternal deprivation.' p. 63. Public Health Paper no. 14. W.H.O. Geneva

Yarrow, L. J. (1961). 'Maternal deprivation: Toward an empirical and conceptual re-evaluation.' *Psychol. Bull.* **58,** 459

Yearbury, E. C. and Newell, N. (1944). 'Genetic and environmental factors in psychoses in children.' *Am. J. Psychiat.* **100,** 599

Youle, W. and Raynes, N. V. (1972). 'Behavioural characteristics of children in residential care in relation to incidence of separation.' *J. Child Psychol. Psychiat.* **13,** 249

INDEX